PUBLIC HEALTH IN THE 21ST CENTURY

UNITED STATES' GLOBAL HEALTH ASSISTANCE

ELEMENTS AND CONSIDERATIONS

Public Health in the 21st Century

Additional books in this series can be found on Nova's website under the Series tab.

Additional e-books in this series can be found on Nova's website under the e-book tab.

PUBLIC HEALTH IN THE 21ST CENTURY

UNITED STATES' GLOBAL HEALTH ASSISTANCE

ELEMENTS AND CONSIDERATIONS

KURK B. WELLER
EDITOR

nova publishers
New York

For permission to use material from this book please contact us:
Telephone 631-231-7269; Fax 631-231-8175
Web Site: http://www.novapublishers.com

NOTICE TO THE READER

Additional color graphics may be available in the e-book version of this book.

Library of Congress Cataloging-in-Publication Data

ISBN: 978-1-62948-387-0

Published by Nova Science Publishers, Inc. † New York

CONTENTS

PREFACE

U.S. support for global health has been motivated in large part by concern about emergent and reemerging infectious diseases. Following outbreaks of diseases like severe acute respiratory syndrome (SARS), HIV/AIDS, and pandemic influenza, several presidents have highlighted the threats they pose to economic development, stability, and security and launched a series of health initiatives to address them. In 1996, for example, President Bill Clinton issued a presidential decision directive that called infectious diseases a threat to domestic and international security and called for U.S. global health efforts to be coordinated with those aimed at counterterrorism. President Clinton later requested $100 million for the Leadership and Investment in Fighting an Epidemic (LIFE) Initiative in 1999 to expand U.S. global HIV/AIDS efforts. President George W. Bush recognized the impact of infectious diseases on domestic and global security in his 2002 and 2006 national security strategy papers and created a number of initiatives aimed at them, including the President's Emergency Plan for AIDS Relief (PEPFAR) in 2004, the President's Malaria Initiative (PMI) in 2005 and the Neglected Tropical Diseases (NTD) Program in 2006. President Barack Obama also recognized the risk of infectious diseases and made several statements about how their spread across developing countries might impact U.S. security. Through the 2010 Quadrennial Diplomacy and Development Review (QDDR) and the 2010 National Security Strategy, the Obama Administration advocated for the coordination of health programs in other areas, such as security, diplomacy and development. Rather than create an initiative aimed at infectious diseases, President Obama sought to address them by affirming U.S. commitment to global health and refining how U.S. global health programs function. In 2009, President Obama announced the Global Health Initiative (GHI), a $63 billion, six-year strategy aimed at improving the coordination and impact of U.S.

global health initiatives. This book provides an overview of global health programs and their effectiveness.

Chapter 1 – Congressional support for global health programs has been increasing, particularly since the George W. Bush Administration. Combined global health funding from State-Foreign Operations, Labor-HHS and Defense appropriations rose from $1.7 billion in FY2001 to $8.9 billion in FY2012. The FY2013 Consolidated Appropriations Act (P.L. 113-6) includes approximately $8.4 billion for global health programs funded through State-Foreign Operations appropriations, up from $8.2 billion in FY2012. (FY2013 funding levels will likely change, however, due to sequestration.) These funds support global health programs implemented and managed by the U.S. Agency for International Development (USAID), State Department and the Global Fund to Fight AIDS, Tuberculosis and Malaria (Global Fund)—a multilateral organization aimed at fighting HIV/AIDS, TB, and malaria worldwide. The act does not specify how much should be spent on global health programs through other appropriations.

Concern about infectious diseases, especially HIV/AIDS, has driven much of the budgetary increases. Excluding funding for the Global Fund, roughly 34% of the FY2001 U.S. global health budget was aimed at programs that address HIV/AIDS. By 2012, about 57% of U.S. global health spending was aimed at fighting HIV/AIDS worldwide, and the FY2014 budget request calls for nearly 54% of global health spending to be aimed at the disease.

In the 112th Congress, concerns about the strength of the U.S. economy and federal spending precipitated discussions about the role and efficacy of U.S. foreign aid, including global health programs. Critics began to push for U.S. global health programs to demonstrate impact and improve cost-efficiency. At the same time, supporters underscored the advances U.S. global health programs had made, the millions of lives saved in part with U.S. resources, and the promise of innovative health solutions. It is likely that this debate will continue in the 113th Congress. Other issues the 113th Congress may face include

- deliberating funding levels for U.S. global health programs;
- examining U.S. leadership of U.S. global health programs;
- maintaining global HIV/AIDS commitments;
- deliberating the reauthorization of the President's Emergency Plan for AIDS Relief (PEPFAR) in FY2013; and
- determining the appropriate mix of multilateral and bilateral spending for global HIV/AIDS, TB, and malaria programs.

These issues are summarized below:

*Global Health Funding***.** Until FY2011, funding for global health had continuously increased. Since then, funding has fluctuated. In FY2011, funding fell slightly and then grew by 0.4% in FY2012. Sequestration requirements are prompting roughly 5% in budget cuts for global health funding in FY2013. In that fiscal year, Congress appropriated nearly $8.5 billion for global health activities funded through State-Foreign Operations, some 8% more than the Administration requested. The FY2014 congressional budget justifications for Labor-HHS and Defense did not specify funding levels for their global health programs. Global health funding will likely be an important issue for the 113th Congress as it considers the FY2014 budget.

GHI Leadership. President Barack Obama created the Global Health Initiative (GHI) to improve the coordination and implementation of U.S. global health programs with the goal of deepening the impact of U.S. global health investments. In the Quadrennial Diplomacy and Development Review, the State Department announced plans to transfer the Office of the Global Health Coordinator from the Department of State to USAID if key milestones were met. In July 2012, the Administration announced that the GHI Office would close, but that the leadership structure for the initiative would be maintained with USAID, the Centers for Disease Control and Prevention (CDC), and the Office of the Global AIDS Coordinator (OGAC) at the State Department collaboratively planning related efforts. At the same time the GHI leadership announced the closing of the GHI Office, the State Department announced the establishment of the Office of Global Health Diplomacy. Some global health observers questioned the rationale for announcing these changes simultaneously.

Maintaining HIV/AIDS Commitments. The Lantos-Hyde Act of 2008 called for the Administration to develop "Partnership Frameworks" with countries that would outline gradual increases in country ownership of PEPFAR programs. As of May 7, 2013, 22 Partnership Frameworks have been signed. Some HIV/AIDS advocates are concerned that these agreements are being prematurely implemented and that countries will not be able to adequately maintain related activities, particularly in the areas of HIV/AIDS treatment. Interruptions in treatment can lead to drug resistance and death. Supporters, however, view these agreements as an important step toward encouraging country ownership and assert that spending reductions are occurring only in countries with a demonstrated capacity to replace the U.S. funds.

PEPFAR Reauthorization. The Lantos-Hyde Act (P.L. 110-293) authorizes appropriations to fight global HIV/AIDS, tuberculosis (TB), and malaria through the Office of the Global AIDS Coordinator (OGAC) and the President's Malaria Initiative (PMI). This act expires at the end of FY2013. If Congress does not reauthorize the legislation, related programs could continue to be funded through annual appropriations, though some language demonstrating congressional intent would expire.

Multilateral and Bilateral Funding. Since the creation of the Global Fund, some debates about U.S. funding for global HIV/AIDS have pitted the Global Fund against PEPFAR. This framing is somewhat inaccurate because U.S. contributions to the Global Fund are part of the PEPFAR budget. Additionally, the Global Fund supports projects aimed at three diseases: HIV/AIDS, TB, and malaria. At the same time, the United States is a key partner of the Global Fund and provides support in a number of areas, including financing, board membership, and collaborative planning. Discussions comparing spending on bilateral HIV/AIDS programs and the Global Fund intensified following an announcement by the Obama Administration that it would seek $4 billion for the Global Fund from FY2011 through FY2013. In FY2010, the Global Fund accounted for 14% of U.S. spending on global HIV/AIDS, TB, and malaria programs. In FY2012, 18% of U.S. funding for the three diseases was directed to the Global Fund. The President requests that in FY2014, 22% of U.S. spending on the three diseases be channeled through the Global Fund.

Although much of the discussions regarding the appropriate mix of multilateral and bilateral funding focus on HIV/AIDS spending, the issue has broader implications for global health programs. According to the World Health Organization (WHO), insufficient alignment of bilateral and multilateral programs is wasteful and inefficient.

Chapter 2 – The President's Emergency Plan for AIDS Relief (PEPFAR) is the largest bilateral health initiative in the world. The 2003 pledge of President George W. Bush to spend $15 billion over five years on fighting HIV/AIDS, tuberculosis (TB), and malaria was considered groundbreaking. The initiative challenged the international community to reject claims that large-scale HIV/AIDS treatment plans could not be carried out in low-resource settings. In December 2002, one month before PEPFAR was announced; only 50,000 people of the estimated 4 million requiring antiretroviral (ARV) medicines in sub-Saharan Africa were receiving treatment. By the end of FY2004, 155,000 people were receiving treatment through PEPFAR.

As of March 2012, PEPFAR has supported

- the provision of anti-retroviral therapy (ART) for more than 4.5 million people (up from 155,000 in 2005);
- testing and counseling for more than 40 million people, including 9.8 million pregnant women;
- prevention of mother-to-child HIV transmission (PMTCT) services for more than 660,000 HIV-positive pregnant women, curbing some 200,000 HIV infections among infants; and
- care and support for more than 13 million people, including more than 4 million orphans and vulnerable children (OVC).

Congress first authorized funds in support of PEPFAR in 2003 through P.L. 108-25, the U.S. Leadership Against HIV/AIDS, Tuberculosis, and Malaria Act (Leadership Act). The $15 billion authorization was to be spent on global HIV/AIDS, TB, and malaria programs from FY2004 through FY2008. Strong bipartisan support for PEPFAR in particular and global health in general led to annual appropriations amounts that exceeded authorized levels. During the first phase of PEPFAR (FY2004-FY2008), the Bush Administration spent $18.1 billion on global HIV/AIDS programs.

As the expiration date of the Leadership Act approached, congressional support for PEPFAR remained enthusiastic. Members debated a range of issues, but ultimately authorized an extension of PEPFAR. The Tom Lantos and Henry J. Hyde United States Global Leadership Against HIV/AIDS, Tuberculosis, and Malaria Reauthorization Act of 2008 (P.L. 110-293, Lantos-Hyde Act) authorized $48 billion to be appropriated from FY2009 through FY2013 for combating the three diseases. From FY2009 through FY2012, the Obama Administration obligated nearly $26 billion on global HIV/AIDS programs.

As the September 30, 2013, expiration date for the authorization of the Lantos-Hyde Act approaches, it is unclear whether Congress will again authorize multiyear funding for PEPFAR. Bipartisan support for PEPFAR remains strong; nonetheless, congressional debate about key elements of the program has raised some concerns. For example, some Members question the extent to which family planning programs are integrated into global HIV/AIDS activities. At the same time, growing unease about the federal budget deficit minimizes the likelihood that past trends of ever-increasing appropriations for global HIV/AIDS programs will be sustained.

Fiscal pressures may have influenced funding amounts that fluctuated (but mostly remained level) throughout the Obama Administration—a departure from the steady growth in spending seen during the Bush Administration. Financial constraints in the global economy have resulted in similar outcomes during the Obama Administration. Whereas many international donors consistently increased their pledges for fighting global HIV/AIDS throughout the Bush Administration, resources made available by key contributors (such as European nations and the Global Fund) began to stagnate and in some cases declined during the past few years. While contributions by traditional donors have mostly stabilized, Brazil, Russia, India, China, and South Africa (BRICS) are playing a greater role in international HIV/AIDS assistance and are transforming from recipient countries into donor nations. At the same time, some aid recipient countries are increasing investments in their own national HIV/AIDS plans.

This report outlines U.S. spending on global HIV/AIDS programs since the inception of PEPFAR, analyzes global HIV/AIDS funding by other donors, and highlights key issues pertaining to funding that will face the 113th Congress as it considers the future of PEPFAR, including

- whether to reauthorize funding for PEPFAR following the expiration of the Lantos-Hyde Act in FY2013;
- engagement with emerging economies and other non-traditional donors who are increasing their participation in the global fight against HIV/AIDS;
- the impact of U.S. efforts to transition ownership of national HIV/AIDS plans to recipient countries;
- the appropriate funding level for the Global Fund;
- whether to support innovative fund-raising approaches for global HIV/AIDS programs, such as taxes on financial transactions and income; and
- developments that might increase HIV/AIDS treatment costs, including intellectual property rights and drug resistance.

Chapter 3 – The Global Fund to Fight AIDS, Tuberculosis, and Malaria (Global Fund, or the Fund) was established in 2002 as a public-private partnership that could provide significant financial support for global responses to HIV/AIDS, tuberculosis (TB), and malaria. By the end of 2011, the Global Fund had approved roughly $22.6 billion to help 150 countries fight these three diseases. According to the Global Fund, from 2002 through

2011, it had supported AIDS treatment for 3.3 million HIV-positive people, anti-tuberculosis treatment for 8.6 million people, and 230 million insecticide-treated nets for the prevention of malaria, saving about 7.7 million lives.

In November 2011, the Global Fund Board announced that due to inadequate resources from donors, it would cancel its 11th round of funding, but would maintain support for existing activities to avoid disruptions in ongoing services. The Fund also announced that it expected to offer new funding for grants in 2014.

The United States has demonstrated strong support for the Global Fund since making a founding pledge in 2001. U.S. officials have served on several Global Fund boards, U.S. contributions to the Fund have surpassed those of any other country, and U.S. global HIV/AIDS, TB, and malaria programs have been increasingly coordinated with Global Fund activities. Donors last met on October 4, 2010, to make their pledges for the Global Fund over the next three years. There, the United States made its first multiyear pledge to the Fund of $4 billion.

Despite rigorous debate on the overall budget and the role of foreign aid in particular, the 112th Congress has maintained support for the Global Fund. In both FY2011 and FY2012, Congress appropriated $1.05 billion for the Global Fund, excluding rescissions. In order to meet the $4 billion multiyear pledge made in 2010, the President's FY2013 budget request included $1.65 billion for the Global Fund, a significant increase from previous years. As part of the budget request, the Administration requested a transfer of $250 million from the State Department's FY2012 bilateral HIV/AIDS funding to the Global Fund, bringing the estimated FY2012 funding level to $1.3 billion.

Global health advocates urge Congress to meet the President's FY2013 request for the Fund in order to support the sustainability of its activities and to encourage continued contributions from other donors. Although Congress has traditionally been a strong supporter of the Fund, several issues may affect congressional views about the Fund in the future. Such factors include the following:

Fiscal austerity. Proposals to reduce federal spending continue to dominate foreign aid debates, with some Members of Congress aiming to target foreign aid accounts, including those for global health, in an attempt to balance the budget. At the same time, others argue that cutting back on the relatively small size of foreign aid (about 1% of total budget authority) will do little to cut the deficit, but could imperil the lives of millions.

Oversight and transparency. In early 2011, reports about misuse of Global Fund resources in some grants ignited a debate about corruption in foreign aid in general, and in the Global Fund in particular. Some have called for donors to withhold support for the Fund until better safeguards are established. Others argue the Fund should not be penalized for oversight shortcomings, which are familiar to many aid programs.

*Role of the Global Fund in U.S. global health policy***.** When the Global Fund was established, U.S. bilateral investments in HIV/AIDS, malaria, and TB were relatively small. Since then, U.S. bilateral investments in fighting these diseases have grown significantly, particularly since the President's Emergency Plan for AIDS Relief (PEPFAR) and the President's Malaria Initiative (PMI) were launched in 2003 and 2005, respectively. Some observers advocate allocating the majority of U.S. funds for global HIV/AIDS and malaria to bilateral programs to ensure sufficient control and oversight of funds. On the other hand, other analysts argue that the Global Fund represents a more efficient and flexible funding mechanism than bilateral programs and offers the United States the ability to pool funds and share risk with other donors, which some believe is particularly important given the challenges of the current fiscal environment.

This report provides background information on the Global Fund, outlines U.S. funding for the Fund, discusses changes the Global Fund has made to improve the efficiency of its programs and address allegations of corruption, and analyzes issues Congress might consider as it debates the appropriate level of U.S support to provide the Fund.

Chapter 4 – In 2010, malaria infected an estimated 216 million people and killed 655,000 people, most of whom were children under the age of five in sub-Saharan Africa. Despite the current burden of disease, malaria is preventable and treatable. Congress has increasingly recognized malaria as an important foreign policy issue, and the United States has become a major player in the global response to the disease. In its second session, the 112th Congress will likely debate the appropriate funding levels and optimum strategy for addressing the continued challenge of global malaria.

Congress has enacted several key pieces of legislation related to global malaria control. These include the Assistance for International Malaria Control Act of 2000 (P.L. 106-570); the U.S. Leadership Against HIV/AIDS, Tuberculosis, and Malaria Act of 2003 (P.L. 108-25); and the Tom Lantos and Henry J. Hyde United States Global Leadership Against HIV/AIDS, Tuberculosis, and Malaria Reauthorization Act of 2008 (P.L. 110-293). These acts have authorized funds to be used in the fight against malaria and have shaped the ways in which U.S. malaria programs are coordinated and managed, including through the creation of the U.S. Global Malaria Coordinator at the United States Agency for International Development (USAID). In 2005, in response to growing international calls for global malaria control and to the success of the President's Emergency Plan for AIDS Relief (PEPFAR), President George W. Bush launched the President's Malaria Initiative (PMI), which aims to halve the burden of malaria morbidity and mortality in 70% of at-risk populations in sub-Saharan Africa by 2014. PMI brought significant new attention and funding to U.S. malaria programs and made the United States one of the largest donors for malaria efforts. While U.S. funding for global malaria programs has increased each fiscal year since FY2004, support for malaria interventions increased most precipitously beginning in FY2007 as PMI has expanded into new countries. President Obama has continued to support PMI through the Global Health Initiative (GHI).

There is evidence that the growing international response to malaria has had some success in controlling the epidemic. Since 2000, global malaria incidence has decreased by 17% and malaria mortality by 26%. Since 2000, 43 countries have reported a reduction in reported malaria cases of more than 50%, including eight African countries that have experienced 50% reduction in either confirmed malaria cases or malaria admissions and deaths. The decreases in each of these African countries are associated with intense malaria control activities. Despite these successes, several key issues pose challenges to an effective scale-up of the response to malaria. First, increasing reports of drug-resistant malaria in Southeast Asia and insecticide-resistant mosquitoes, largely in Africa, threaten the success of malaria control programs. Second, weak health systems, including shortages in health care personnel and inadequate supply chain networks, have limited the delivery of essential commodities for malaria control. There is also debate within the global health community over whether malaria efforts should increasingly target areas where malaria elimination is possible or whether efforts should remain concentrated on malaria control.

This report outlines basic facts related to global malaria, including characteristics of the epidemic and U.S. legislation, programs, funding, and partnerships related to the global response to malaria.

Chapter 5 – The term "neglected tropical diseases" (NTDs) was coined by the World Health Organization (WHO) in 2003 to describe a set of diseases that are ancient, worsen poverty, and typically impair health and productivity while carrying low death rates. Some NTDs are easily treatable; others are not.

While the use of the term "NTDs" has helped to raise awareness about these longstanding health challenges, its use risks simplifying a complicated health challenge. Health interventions to address the array of NTDs vary, but a common factor to an enduring solution to these illnesses is economic development. Industrialized countries, including the United States, have controlled these diseases in their territories by combining drug treatment with the construction and use of improved sanitation, modernization of agricultural practices, and utilization of improved water systems. Neglected tropical diseases are diseases that primarily plague the poorest people in developing countries. Changes in the environment and population flows, however, make industrialized countries, including the United States, increasingly vulnerable to some NTDs, particularly dengue haemorrhagic fever, for which there is no cure.

Congressional interest in NTDs has been growing. Appropriations for NTD programs have steadily increased from $15 million in FY2006 to $89 million in FY2012. The Administration requested $67 million to support NTD programs in FY2013. In addition to raising spending for NTDs, Congress has taken other actions to demonstrate support for tackling NTDs. In October 2009, for example, the House Malaria Caucus expanded its purview to include NTDs. The Senate Malaria Caucus did the same in September 2012.

The international community has made substantial progress in combating select NTDs, though some have been tackled more effectively than others. Guinea worm disease, for example, is on the cusp of eradication.

More generally, expanding access to mass drug administration is contributing to decreases in prevalence of several NTDs, particularly across Latin America. Despite these advances, WHO cautions that these diseases cannot be banished without improving global access to clean water and sanitation, strengthening local health capacity (veterinary as well as human), and intensifying case detection and management. Making improvements in these areas will require long-term investments that are complex and may entail facing thorny issues such as addressing corruption, transferring ownership of health programs from donors to recipient countries, and evaluating the impact of political and economic policies on health programs (e.g., international lending requirements).

The United States has played an important role in combating NTDs, and President Barack Obama has prioritized tackling NTDs. Recommendations for congressional action may largely reflect broader arguments about congressional engagement in improving global health. Analysts who support congressional directives that set programmatic targets, outline the types of activities to be implemented in U.S. global health programs, and mandate reporting requirements would probably argue for the 113th Congress to take similar steps. Observers who maintain that these steps make U.S. global health programs less effective by minimizing the capacity of implementing agencies to adapt global health programs to local conditions would likely argue for limiting congressional support for combating NTDs to appropriating sufficient resources. This report discusses the prevalence of NTDs, U.S. and global actions to address them, and options the 113th Congress might consider.

In: United States' Global Health Assistance
Editors: Kurk B. Weller
ISBN: 978-1-62948-387-0

Chapter 1

U.S. GLOBAL HEALTH ASSISTANCE: BACKGROUND AND ISSUES FOR THE 113TH CONGRESS*

Tiaji Salaam-Blyther

SUMMARY

Congressional support for global health programs has been increasing, particularly since the George W. Bush Administration. Combined global health funding from State-Foreign Operations, Labor-HHS and Defense appropriations rose from $1.7 billion in FY2001 to $8.9 billion in FY2012. The FY2013 Consolidated Appropriations Act (P.L. 113-6) includes approximately $8.4 billion for global health programs funded through State-Foreign Operations appropriations, up from $8.2 billion in FY2012. (FY2013 funding levels will likely change, however, due to sequestration.) These funds support global health programs implemented and managed by the U.S. Agency for International Development (USAID), State Department and the Global Fund to Fight AIDS, Tuberculosis and Malaria (Global Fund)—a multilateral organization aimed at fighting HIV/AIDS, TB, and malaria worldwide. The act does not specify how much should be spent on global health programs through other appropriations.

* This is an edited, reformatted and augmented version of a Congressional Research Service publication, CRS Report for Congress R43115, prepared for Members and Committees of Congress, from www.crs.gov, dated June 21, 2013.

Concern about infectious diseases, especially HIV/AIDS, has driven much of the budgetary increases. Excluding funding for the Global Fund, roughly 34% of the FY2001 U.S. global health budget was aimed at programs that address HIV/AIDS. By 2012, about 57% of U.S. global health spending was aimed at fighting HIV/AIDS worldwide, and the FY2014 budget request calls for nearly 54% of global health spending to be aimed at the disease.

In the 112th Congress, concerns about the strength of the U.S. economy and federal spending precipitated discussions about the role and efficacy of U.S. foreign aid, including global health programs. Critics began to push for U.S. global health programs to demonstrate impact and improve cost-efficiency. At the same time, supporters underscored the advances U.S. global health programs had made, the millions of lives saved in part with U.S. resources, and the promise of innovative health solutions. It is likely that this debate will continue in the 113th Congress. Other issues the 113th Congress may face include

- deliberating funding levels for U.S. global health programs;
- examining U.S. leadership of U.S. global health programs;
- maintaining global HIV/AIDS commitments;
- deliberating the reauthorization of the President's Emergency Plan for AIDS Relief (PEPFAR) in FY2013; and
- determining the appropriate mix of multilateral and bilateral spending for global HIV/AIDS, TB, and malaria programs.

These issues are summarized below.

*Global Health Funding***.** Until FY2011, funding for global health had continuously increased. Since then, funding has fluctuated. In FY2011, funding fell slightly and then grew by 0.4% in FY2012. Sequestration requirements are prompting roughly 5% in budget cuts for global health funding in FY2013. In that fiscal year, Congress appropriated nearly $8.5 billion for global health activities funded through State-Foreign Operations, some 8% more than the Administration requested. The FY2014 congressional budget justifications for Labor-HHS and Defense did not specify funding levels for their global health programs. Global health funding will likely be an important issue for the 113th Congress as it considers the FY2014 budget.

GHI Leadership. President Barack Obama created the Global Health Initiative (GHI) to improve the coordination and implementation of U.S. global health programs with the goal of deepening the impact of U.S. global health investments. In the Quadrennial Diplomacy and Development Review, the State Department announced plans to transfer the Office of the Global Health Coordinator from the Department of State to USAID if key milestones were met. In July 2012, the Administration announced that the GHI Office would close, but that the leadership structure for the initiative would be maintained with USAID, the Centers for Disease Control and Prevention (CDC), and the Office of the Global AIDS Coordinator (OGAC) at the State Department collaboratively planning related efforts. At the same time the GHI leadership announced the closing of the GHI Office, the State Department announced the establishment of the Office of Global Health Diplomacy. Some global health observers questioned the rationale for announcing these changes simultaneously.

Maintaining HIV/AIDS Commitments. The Lantos-Hyde Act of 2008 called for the Administration to develop "Partnership Frameworks" with countries that would outline gradual increases in country ownership of PEPFAR programs. As of May 7, 2013, 22 Partnership Frameworks have been signed. Some HIV/AIDS advocates are concerned that these agreements are being prematurely implemented and that countries will not be able to adequately maintain related activities, particularly in the areas of HIV/AIDS treatment. Interruptions in treatment can lead to drug resistance and death. Supporters, however, view these agreements as an important step toward encouraging country ownership and assert that spending reductions are occurring only in countries with a demonstrated capacity to replace the U.S. funds.

PEPFAR Reauthorization. The Lantos-Hyde Act (P.L. 110-293) authorizes appropriations to fight global HIV/AIDS, tuberculosis (TB), and malaria through the Office of the Global AIDS Coordinator (OGAC) and the President's Malaria Initiative (PMI). This act expires at the end of FY2013. If Congress does not reauthorize the legislation, related programs could continue to be funded through annual appropriations, though some language demonstrating congressional intent would expire.

Multilateral and Bilateral Funding. Since the creation of the Global Fund, some debates about U.S. funding for global HIV/AIDS have pitted the Global Fund against PEPFAR. This framing is somewhat inaccurate because U.S. contributions to the Global Fund are part of the PEPFAR budget. Additionally, the Global Fund supports projects aimed at three diseases: HIV/AIDS, TB, and malaria. At the same time, the United States is a key partner of the Global Fund and provides support in a number of areas, including financing, board membership, and collaborative planning. Discussions comparing spending on bilateral HIV/AIDS programs and the Global Fund intensified following an announcement by the Obama Administration that it would seek $4 billion for the Global Fund from FY2011 through FY2013. In FY2010, the Global Fund accounted for 14% of U.S. spending on global HIV/AIDS, TB, and malaria programs. In FY2012, 18% of U.S. funding for the three diseases was directed to the Global Fund. The President requests that in FY2014, 22% of U.S. spending on the three diseases be channeled through the Global Fund.

Although much of the discussions regarding the appropriate mix of multilateral and bilateral funding focus on HIV/AIDS spending, the issue has broader implications for global health programs. According to the World Health Organization (WHO), insufficient alignment of bilateral and multilateral programs is wasteful and inefficient.

INTRODUCTION

Congress has demonstrated interest in global health and has generally appropriated funds for global health in excess of presidential requests, particularly since FY2000. U.S. government funding for global health has grown from $1.7 billion in FY2001 to $8.9 billion in FY2012 (*Figure 1*). The Administration proposes spending more than $9 billion on global health programs in FY2014.

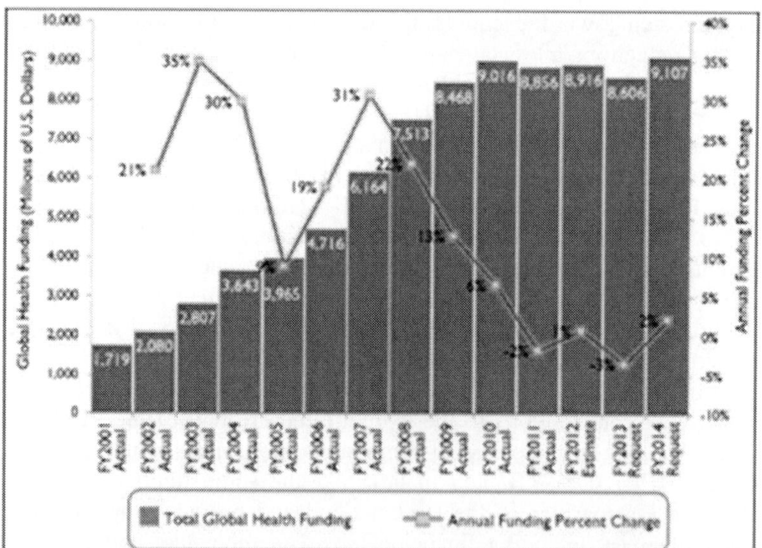

Source: Created by CRS from appropriations legislation and data received from the Office of Management and Budget (OMB).

Note: Includes global health funding through three appropriations vehicles: State-Foreign Operations; Labor, HHS, and Education (Labor-HHS); and Defense. HIV/AIDS amounts include U.S. contributions to the Global Fund to Fight AIDS, Tuberculosis and Malaria.

Figure 1. U.S. Global Health Funding: FY2001-FY2014 Request. (current U.S. millions of dollars).

- U.S. support for global health has been motivated in large part by concern about emergent and reemerging infectious diseases. Following outbreaks of diseases like severe acute respiratory syndrome (SARS), HIV/AIDS, and pandemic influenza, several presidents have highlighted the threats they pose to economic development, stability, and security and launched a series of health initiatives to address them. In 1996, for example, President Bill Clinton issued a presidential decision directive that called infectious diseases a threat to domestic and international security and called for U.S. global health efforts to be coordinated with those aimed at counterterrorism.[1]
- President Clinton later requested $100 million for the Leadership and Investment in Fighting an Epidemic (LIFE) Initiative in 1999 to expand U.S. global HIV/AIDS efforts.[2] President George W. Bush recognized the impact of infectious diseases on domestic and global security in his 2002 and 2006 national security strategy papers and created a number of initiatives aimed at them, including the President's Emergency Plan for AIDS Relief (PEPFAR) in 2004, the President's Malaria Initiative (PMI) in 2005 and the Neglected Tropical Diseases (NTD) Program in 2006.[3]
- President Barack Obama also recognized the risk of infectious diseases and made several statements about how their spread across developing countries might impact U.S. security.[4] Through the 2010 Quadrennial Diplomacy and Development Review (QDDR) and the 2010 National Security Strategy, the Obama Administration advocated for the coordination of health programs in other areas, such as security, diplomacy and development. Rather than create an initiative aimed at infectious diseases, President Obama sought to address them by affirming U.S. commitment to global health and refining how U.S. global health programs function. In 2009, President Obama announced the Global Health Initiative (GHI), a $63 billion, six-year strategy aimed at improving the coordination and impact of U.S. global health initiatives (described fully in the section entitled, "The Global Health Initiative (GHI)").
- Legislative and executive branch support for raising global health budgets have been largely aligned, though some debates have emerged on more finite issues, such as the type of HIV/AIDS interventions to support. Recurring debate has also centered on international family planning and reproductive health programs.[5]

During the 112th Congress, concerns about slow economic recovery began to erode support for maintaining higher global health spending levels. Some Members questioned levels of non-security foreign aid and argued for the reduction or elimination of development and health assistance. In total, foreign aid accounts for less than 1% of the federal budget. Some Members contended cuts to these programs could yield important savings, while others maintained such reductions would have little impact on the federal deficit, could imperil the lives of vulnerable populations reliant on U.S. assistance, and might erode progress achieved through increased investments. Examples of progress in global health aid include the following:

Debates about U.S. global health funding levels will likely continue in the 113th Congress and may intensify as Members seek to reduce overall spending.

APPROPRIATIONS FOR U.S. GLOBAL HEALTH PROGRAMS

Congress funds most global health assistance through three appropriations bills: State-Foreign Operations and Related Programs (State-Foreign Operations); Labor, Health and Human Services, and Education (Labor-HHS); and Department of Defense (*Figure 2*). These bills are used to fund global health efforts implemented by USAID, CDC, and the Department of Defense (DOD), including PEPFAR programs that are coordinated by the Department of State and implemented by several U.S. agencies (*Figure 3*). Through PEPFAR, the United States contributes to multilateral efforts to combat HIV/AIDS, TB, and malaria, including the Global Fund and the Joint United Nations Program on HIV/AIDS (UNAIDS).

Reports about U.S. spending on global health can vary because there is no single "global health" appropriation. Some groups count funding for development issues that impact health, like water and sanitation, towards U.S. global health spending. This report focuses on activities that receive a specific amount for global health through State-Foreign Operations appropriations and Labor-HHS appropriations, and for global HIV/AIDS through Department of Defense appropriations. Specific activities supported through these three appropriations vehicles are discussed below.

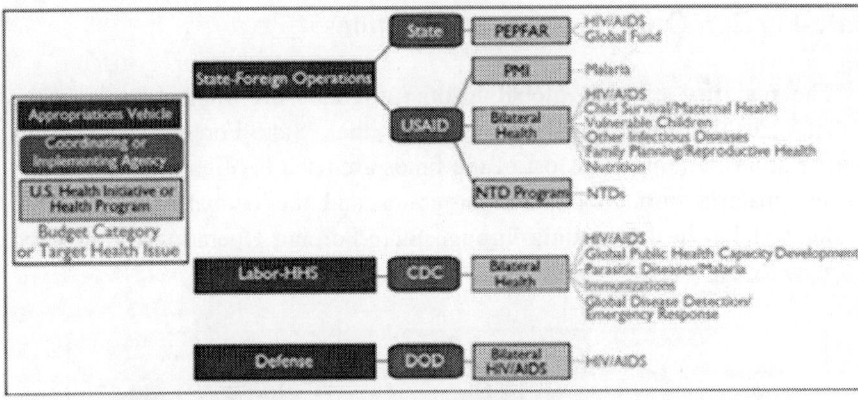

Source: Created by CRS from appropriations legislation.

Figure 2. U.S. Global Health Assistance: Appropriation Vehicles.

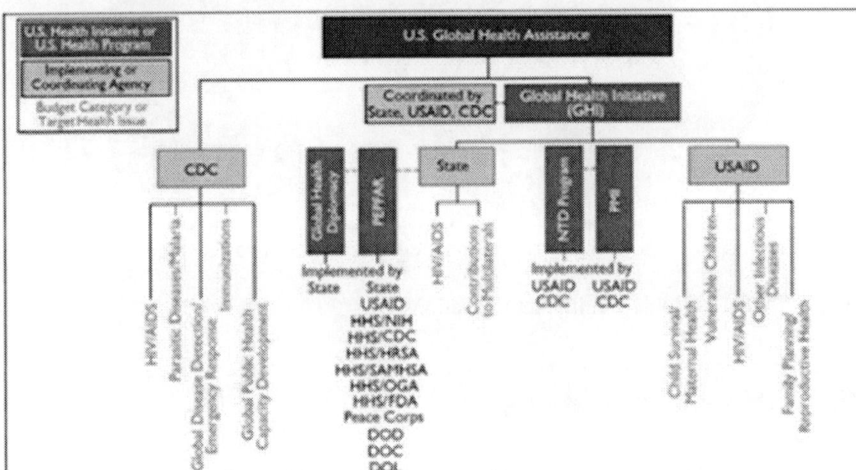

Source: Created by CRS from appropriations legislation.

Notes: Appropriations for HIV/AIDS programs implemented by CDC, State and USAID are part of PEPFAR.

Acronyms not previously described: Department of Commerce (DOC), Department of Labor (DOL), Department of State (State), Food and Drug Administration (FDA), Health Resources and Services Administration (HRSA), National Institutes of Health (NIH) Office of Global Health Affairs, Substance Abuse and Mental Health Services Administration (SAMHSA).

Figure 3. U.S. Global Health Assistance: Implementing Agencies and Initiatives.

State-Foreign Operations Appropriations

The majority of U.S. global health programs are funded through the Global Health Programs Account in the State-Foreign Operations appropriations (*Figure 4*). Most of the funds are used for fighting HIV/AIDS, TB and malaria through bilateral programs and the Global Fund. A table outlining global health funding through State-Foreign Operations is included in *Appendix C.*

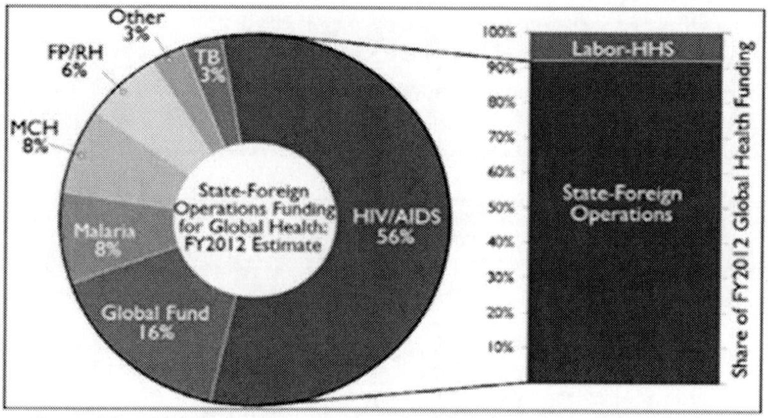

Source: Created by CRS from appropriations legislation and data received from OMB.

Figure 4. FY2012 Global Health Appropriations.

Labor-HHS Appropriations

Through Labor-HHS appropriations, Congress funds global health programs implemented by CDC and provides resources to support international HIV/AIDS research conducted by the National Institutes of Health (NIH). Congress appropriates specific amounts for various global health programs implemented by CDC, though the appropriations language does not cover the breadth of global health activities managed by CDC. At the same time, appropriations language does not specify a particular amount for global HIV/AIDS research grants funded through NIH, though the Administration typically includes these amounts in reports on PEPFAR funding. A table outlining global health spending through Labor-HHS is included in *Appendix C.*

Defense Appropriations

Congress appropriates funds to DOD in support of its PEPFAR-related work through Defense appropriations. On average, Congress provides between $8 million and $10 million annually for these purposes. At the same time, DOD receives additional resources from the State Department as an implementing partner of PEPFAR. A table outlining U.S. funding for global HIV/AIDS programs, including those implemented by DOD, is included in *Appendix C*.

IMPLEMENTING AGENCIES AND DEPARTMENTS

This section briefly describes global health activities implemented or coordinated by each agency or department with appropriations, as described above. This discussion is limited to those agencies and departments for which Congress provides specific funding: USAID, State, CDC, and DOD.

U.S. Agency for International Development[14]

USAID groups its global health activities into three areas: saving mothers and children, creating an AIDS-Free generation, and fighting other infectious diseases. A summary of these efforts is described below.

- *Saving Mothers and Children.* USAID seeks to save the lives of women and children by reducing morbidity and mortality from common diseases and under nutrition; supporting vulnerable children and orphans; increasing access to family planning; and raising awareness about reproductive health. Under this category, Congress designates a specific amount for the following health areas:
  - maternal and child health,
  - malaria,
  - nutrition,
  - family planning and reproductive health, and
  - social services (vulnerable children).

- *Creating an AIDS-Free Generation.* USAID aims to combat HIV/AIDS by supporting voluntary counseling and testing, awareness campaigns, and the supply of antiretroviral medicines, among other activities.
- *Fighting Other Infectious Diseases.* USAID works to address a number of infectious diseases and resultant outbreaks. Congress appropriates a specific amount for: TB, pandemic influenza and other emerging threats, and NTDs.

Centers for Disease Control and Prevention[15]

Through Labor-HHS appropriations, Congress specifies support for the following CDC global health activities:

- *HIV/AIDS.* CDC works with Ministries of Health (MOHs) and global partners to increase access to integrated HIV/AIDS care and treatment services; strengthen and expand high-quality laboratory services; conduct research; and support resource-constrained countries develop sustainable public health systems.
- *Parasitic Diseases and Malaria.* CDC aims to reduce death and illness associated with parasitic diseases, including malaria, by capacity building and enhancing surveillance, monitoring and evaluation, vector control, case management, and diagnostic testing. CDC also identifies best practices for parasitic disease programs and conducts epidemiological and laboratory research for the development of new tools and strategies.
- *Global Disease Detection (GDD) and Emergency Response.* Through GDD, CDC builds capacity to monitor, detect, and assess disease threats and responds to requests from other U.S. agencies, United Nations agencies, and nongovernmental organizations for support in humanitarian assistance activities.
- *Global Immunization.* CDC works to advance several global immunization initiatives aimed at preventable diseases, including polio, measles, rubella, and meningitis; accelerate the introduction of new vaccines; and strengthen immunization systems in priority countries through technical assistance, monitoring and evaluation, social mobilization and vaccine management.

- *Global Public Health Capacity Development.* CDC help MOHs develop Field Epidemiology Training Programs (FETPs) that strengthen health systems by enhancing laboratory management, applied research, communications, program evaluation, program management, and disease detection and response.

Department of State

Through OGAC, the State Department leads PEPFAR and oversees all U.S. spending on global HIV/AIDS, including those appropriated to other agencies and multilateral groups like the Global Fund and UNAIDS. In July 2012, the Administration announced an expansion of the State Department's engagement in global health with the launch of the Office of Global Health Diplomacy (OGHD).[16] The office seeks to "guide diplomatic efforts to advance the United States' global health mission" and provide "diplomatic support in implementing the Global Health Initiative's principles and goals."[17] The Global AIDS Coordinator also leads OGHD. The key objectives of the OGHD are to

- provide ambassadors with expertise, support and tools to help them effectively work with country officials on global health issues;
- elevate the role of ambassadors in their efforts to pursue diplomatic strategies and partnerships within countries to advance health;
- support ambassadors to build political will among partner countries to improve health and strengthen health systems;
- strengthen the sustainability of health programs by helping partner countries meet the health care needs of their own people and achieve country ownership; and
- foster shared responsibility and coordination among donor nations, multilateral institutions, civil society, the private sector, faith-based organizations, foundations, and community members.

Following the announcement of the OGHD, some observers questioned whether the Administration was quietly abandoning GHI. For more on this issue, see section on "Coordinating GHI."

Department of Defense

DOD carries out a wide range of health activities abroad, including infectious disease research, health assistance following natural disasters and other emergencies, and training of foreign health workers and officials.[18] The only global health activity for which Congress provides a specific appropriation, however, is DOD's HIV/AIDS Prevention Program (DHAAP). Congress has never appropriated more than $10 million to DOD for its global HIV/AIDS work, though it receives transfers from the Department of State as an implementing agency of PEPFAR. These funds are used to support research, care, treatment and prevention programs.[19] *Table C-4* in *Appendix C* outlines annual funding for DHAAP.

U.S. Government Global Health Initiatives

As previously discussed, Presidents Clinton and Bush created global health initiatives to address infectious diseases (*Figure 5).* During the Bush Administration, consensus emerged that these initiatives, particularly PEPFAR, needed to be better integrated with other public health activities to improve efficiency and sustainability. President Obama maintained support for the Bush Era health initiatives but attempted to address these concerns with the launch of the GHI. The section below describes these global health initiatives.

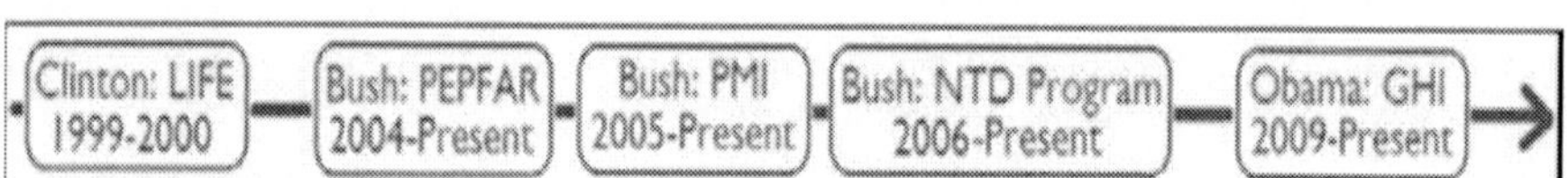
Clinton: LIFE
1999-2000
Bush: PEPFAR
2004-Present
Bush: PMI
2005-Present
Bush: NTD Program
2006-Present
Obama: GHI
2009-Present

Source: Created by CRS.

Figure 5. Timeline of U.S. Government Global Health Initiatives.

President's Emergency Plan for AIDS Relief (PEPFAR)[20]

In January 2003, President Bush announced PEPFAR, a government-wide initiative to combat global HIV/AIDS. PEPFAR supports a wide range of HIV/AIDS prevention, treatment, and care activities and is the largest commitment by any nation to combat a single disease. Later that year, Congress enacted the Leadership Act (P.L. 108-25), which authorized $15 billion to be spent from FY2004-FY2008 on bilateral and multilateral

HIV/AIDS, TB and malaria programs and authorized the creation of OGAC to oversee all U.S. spending on global HIV/AIDS. OGAC distributes the majority of the funds it receives from Congress for global HIV/AIDS programs to multilateral groups like the Global Fund, as well as federal agencies and departments. In 2008, Congress enacted the Lantos-Hyde Act (P.L. 110-293), which authorized the appropriation of $48 billion for global HIV/AIDS, TB, and malaria efforts from FY2009-FY2013.

President's Malaria Initiative (PMI)[21]

In June 2005, President Bush announced PMI to expand and coordinate U.S. global malaria efforts. PMI was originally established as a five-year, $1.2 billion effort to halve the number of malaria-related deaths in 15 sub-Saharan African countries through the expansion of four prevention and treatment techniques: indoor residual spraying (IRS), insecticide-treated nets (ITNs), artemisinin-based combination therapies (ACTs), and intermittent preventative treatment for pregnant women (IPTp).[22] The Obama Administration expanded the goals of PMI to halving the burden of malaria among 70% of at-risk populations in Africa by 2014 and added the Democratic Republic of Congo, Guinea, Nigeria, and Zimbabwe as partner countries.

The Lantos-Hyde Act authorized the establishment of the U.S. Malaria Coordinator at USAID. The Malaria Coordinator oversees implementation efforts of USAID and CDC and is advised by an Interagency Advisory Group that includes representatives from USAID, HHS, State, DOD, the National Security Council (NSC), and the Office of Management and Budget (OMB).

Neglected Tropical Disease (NTD) Program[23]

The NTD Program started in 2006, following FY2006 appropriations language that directed USAID to make available at least $15 million for fighting seven NTDs.[24] It is managed by USAID and jointly implemented by USAID and CDC. When the program was launched, the Bush Administration sought to support the provision of 160 million NTD treatments for 40 million people in 15 countries. In 2008, President Bush reaffirmed his commitment to tackling NTDs and proposed spending $350 million from FY2008 through FY2013 on expanding the program to 30 countries. In 2009, the Obama Administration amended the targets of the NTD program and called for the

United States to support halving the prevalence of NTDs among 70% of the affected population in target countries.

The Global Health Initiative (GHI)

In May 2009, President Obama announced GHI to expand the impact of U.S. government health programs. GHI aims to improve the coordination and integration of U.S. bilateral global health programs, which were described above, and emphasizes the application of results-based funding. Other important goals of GHI include the following:

- increasing the impact of U.S. global health investments;
- advancing country ownership of health aid;
- strengthening health systems;
- investing in women and girls; and
- enhancing program monitoring and evaluation and research and innovation.[25]

GHI encompasses global health activities implemented by USAID and carried out through PEPFAR and PMI. The initiative aims to advance sustainable improvements in global health in three areas: protecting communities from infectious diseases, saving the lives of mothers and children and creating an AIDS-free generation. In each of these areas, the Administration has set goals and measurable indicators. For a description of these, see *Figure A-1* in *Appendix A*.

Through GHI, the U.S. government is developing "country strategies" that outline U.S. support for national health plans. The purpose of the strategies is to align the goals of GHI and partner countries, coordinate U.S. global health efforts, and enhance the efficiency and sustainability of these efforts. The strategies are developed in the U.S. missions by representatives of each implementing agency and have reportedly been completed for approximately 40 countries.[26] As of June 18, 2013, GHI has published 35 of these (*Figure 6)*.

Coordinating GHI

From 2011 to mid-2012, GHI was coordinated by an executive director at the Department of State who reported to the Secretary of State and the GHI Operations Committee.

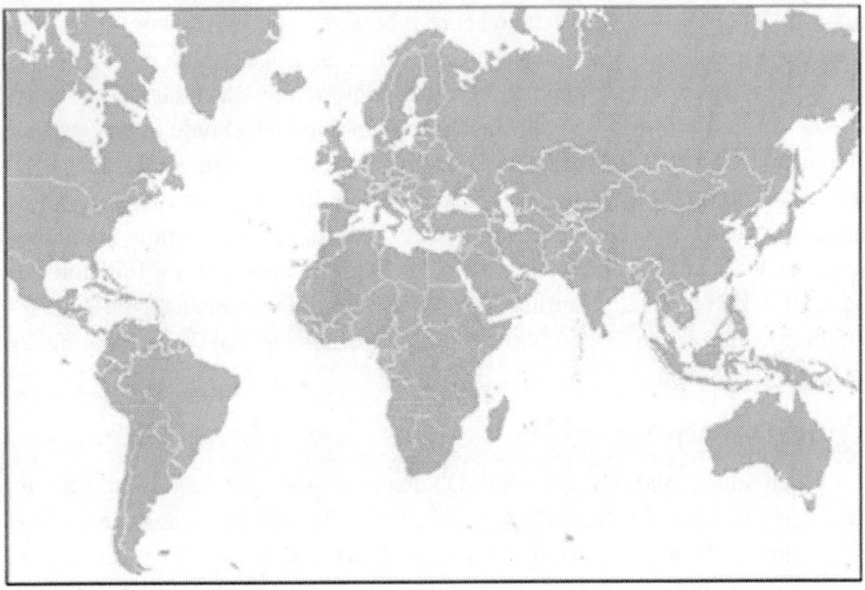

Source: GHI website, http://www.ghi.gov/country/index.htm, accessed on June 18, 2013.

Notes: The country strategies have been published for Armenia, Bangladesh, Benin, Bolivia, Burundi, Cambodia, Democratic Republic of Congo, Dominican Republic, Ethiopia, Georgia, Ghana, Guatemala, Honduras, Indonesia, Kenya, Lesotho, Liberia, Malawi, Mali, Mozambique, Namibia, Nepal, Nigeria, Philippines, Rwanda, Senegal, Sierra Leone, South Africa, Swaziland, Tanzania, Uganda, Ukraine, Vietnam, Zambia, and Zimbabwe.

Figure 6. GHI Country Strategies: A Map.

The committee, which oversees and manages GHI, is chaired by the USAID Administrator, the Global AIDS Coordinator, and the Director of CDC. The Administration considered transferring leadership of GHI from the State Department to USAID by late FY2012 on the condition that USAID met a set of benchmarks related to management capacity, as outlined in the Quadrennial Diplomacy and Development Review (QDDR).[27]

In July 2012, the co-coordinators of GHI—Ambassador Goosby (State/OGAC), Lois Quam (State/GHI), Administrator Rajiv Shah (USAID) and Director Thomas Frieden (CDC)— announced a collective recommendation to end the QDDR benchmark process, close the GHI office, and establish an Office of Global Health Diplomacy (GHD) at the Department of State to guide diplomatic efforts for advancing the U.S. global health mission.[28] The press release underscored, however, that GHI would continue to be the central focus and guiding strategy of U.S. global health programs.

Several observers debated the implications of the statement, particularly whether the Administration was quietly abandoning GHI. Some interpreted the announcement as a signal that the Administration was using the new GHD office to indirectly resolve arguments in Washington about who should ultimately lead U.S. global health efforts.[29] The Administration maintains, however, that the GHD office is not taking over the coordinating function that the GHI office played.[30] Further, the Administration maintains a website for GHI and continues to cite it as the guiding mechanism for U.S. global health work.

Funding GHI

When launching GHI, President Obama proposed spending $63 billion on global health from FY2009 through FY2014. The President announced that $51 billion of those funds would be aimed at HIV/AIDS and TB programs and the rest on global health programs implemented by USAID. From FY2009-FY2012, GHI funding reached $34.3 billion. The FY2013 Consolidated Appropriations act provided an additional $5.7 billion for State-managed HIV/AIDS programs, including $1.65 billion for the Global Fund. The act also included nearly $2.8 billion for global health programs implemented by USAID, though it did not specify for which programs. *Figure 7* estimates the additional funds needed to meet the GHI funding goals. This figure will likely change, however, as FY2013 funding levels for global health spending under sequestration has not yet been released.

HIV/AIDS, TB and Malaria Programs. From FY2009-FY2012, the United States spent $34.3 billion on global HIV/AIDS, TB and malaria programs. The FY2013 Consolidated Appropriations act appropriated $5.7 billion for State-managed HIV/AIDS programs, including $1.65 billion for the Global Fund. Assuming that other HIV/AIDS, TB and malaria-related efforts are funded at FY2012 levels in FY2013 and that the President's FY2014 budget for the diseases is met, funding for fighting these three diseases would be roughly $7 billion—or—about 15% less than sought by the Administration, though this amount may change following sequestration.

Non-HIV/AIDS, TB and Malaria Programs. From FY2009-FY2012, the United States spent nearly $5.2 billion on non-HIV/AIDS, TB and malaria programs. The FY2013 Consolidated Appropriations act appropriated almost $2.8 billion for global health programs implemented by USAID. Assuming that USAID's HIV/AIDS, TB and malaria programs would be funded at

FY2012 levels for FY2013 and that the President's FY2014 budget for other health programs is met, funding for programs not associated with these three diseases would be about $5.2 billion— or some 32%—less than sought by the Administration, though this amount may change following sequestration.

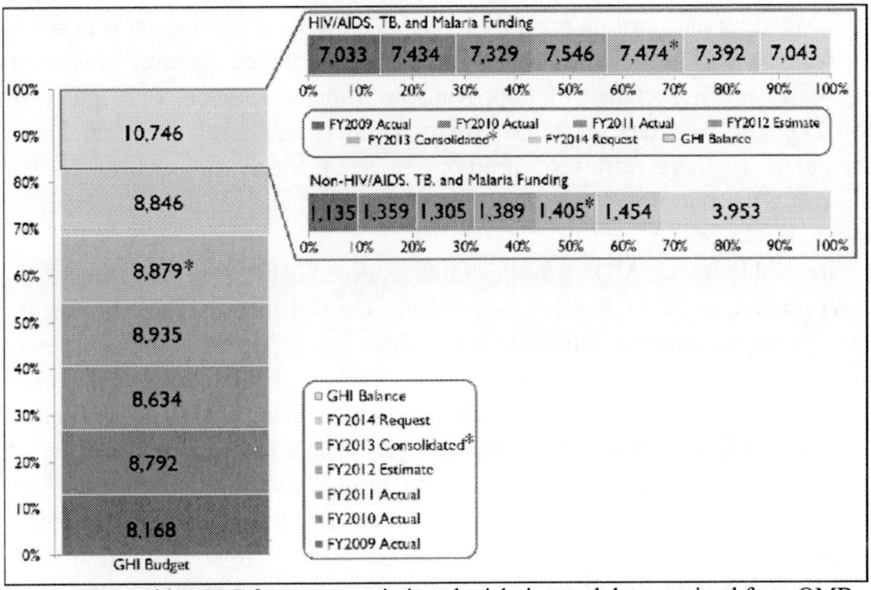

Source: Created by CRS from appropriations legislation and data received from OMB.

Notes: *FY2013 HIV/AIDS, TB, and malaria total was calculated by adding the $4.1 billion for State-HIV/AIDS and $1.65 for the Global Fund, as specified in the FY2013 Consolidated Appropriations act with FY2012 estimates for related programs. These include $350 million for USAID HIV/AIDS programs, $650 million for USAID malaria programs, $236 million for USAID TB programs, $117.8 million for CDC HIV/AIDS programs, $9.4 million for CDC malaria programs, and 8.0 million for DOD HIV/AIDS programs. The $388.9 million FY2013 request is used for NIH international HIV/AIDS research, as the Administration's request is generally met and Congress does not provide an amount for this program. Instead, NIH draws the funds from the budget for the Office of HIV/AIDS Research. Due to sequestration, however, these figures will likely change.

Figure 7. GHI Funding: FY2009-FY2014. (current U.S. millions and percentage of GHI budget goal).

Prioritizing Non-HIV/AIDS Programs Through GHI

One goal of GHI is to improve the health of women and children, particularly through investments in maternal and child health, family planning and reproductive health and nutrition. The President also seeks to increase support for fighting other infectious diseases like NTDs. Congress has supported these ideas and increased funding in these areas. From FY2009 through FY2012, funding for maternal and child health grew by 22% and rose by 15% for family planning and reproductive health. During the same time period funding for nutrition grew by 73% and more than doubled for NTDs.

Nutrition. The Obama Administration has taken several steps to emphasize the importance of improving nutrition worldwide. In September 2010, former Secretary of State Hillary Clinton launched the 1,000 Days Campaign, a global effort to promote targeted action and investment in improving the nutritional status of pregnant women and children within their first two years of life.[31]

In addition, USAID Administrator Rajiv Shah serves as the U.S. representative to the United Nations Scaling Up Nutrition (SUN) Movement, which aims to improve nutrition worldwide.[32] A group of Nobel Laureate economic experts ranked efforts to address undernutrition as the most cost-effective investment in foreign aid. The economists concluded that each dollar spent on reducing chronic undernutrition could yield a $30 benefit.[33]

The Administration addresses nutrition through a variety of programs. For example, nutrition is a link between the Global Health Initiative and the Feed the Future (FtF) Initiative. Focus countries for FtF are largely aligned around GHI countries with the highest burden of undernutrition. USAID also uses resources through accounts like the Development Assistance account and McGovern-Dole International Food for Education to improve nutrition worldwide, though funding levels for nutrition activities within these accounts are not set by Congress. USAID is reportedly working on a strategic framework that would improve means for tracking nutrition funding and outcomes across all programs, especially global health, food security and food aid.

Other Infectious Diseases. President Obama has advocated increasing funding for programs to combat other infectious diseases. Congressional support for this idea preceded the GHI. From FY2000-FY2012 funding grew for TB by 45% and malaria by 70%. From FY2006-FY2012, funding rose by 256% for NTDs. Despite these increases, TB and NTD programs continued to account for less than 3% and 2% of the GHI budget respectively due to the large portion of the budget aimed at the HIV/AIDS and the Global Fund (*Figure 8*).

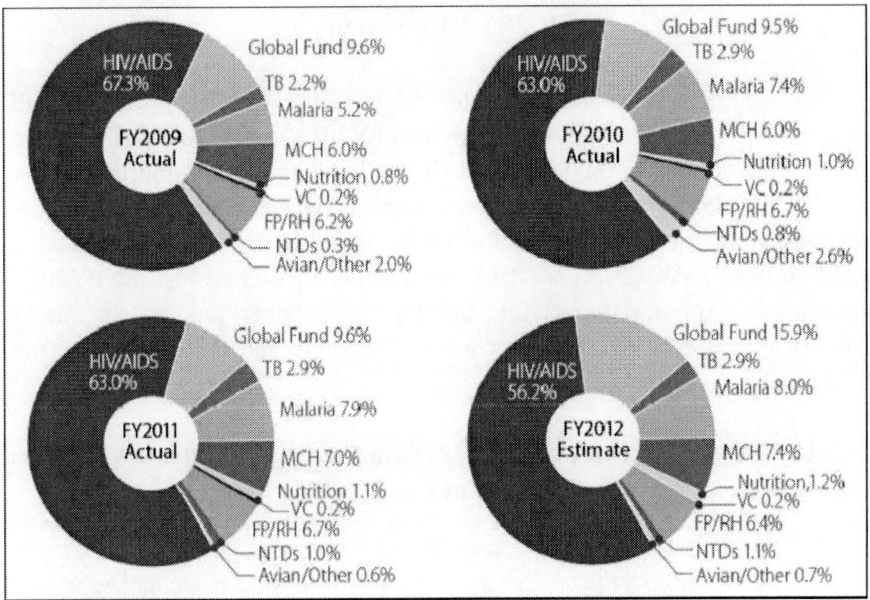

Source: Created by CRS from appropriations legislation and data received from OMB.

Abbreviations: Maternal and Child Health (MCH), Vulnerable Children (VC), Tuberculosis (TB), Family Planning and Reproductive Health (FP/RH), Neglected Tropical Diseases (NTDs).

Figure 8. GHI Global Health Spending, by Program Area, FY2009-FY2012. (in millions of current U.S. dollars and percentages).

Non-Communicable Diseases. The majority of U.S. global health resources are aimed at fighting infectious diseases. Nonetheless, non-communicable diseases (NCDs) are a growing problem in middle-income and developing countries. More than 36 million people died from NCDs worldwide in 2008, primarily from cardiovascular diseases (CVDs), which accounted for 48% of NCD deaths. Some 21% of NCD deaths were attributable to cancers, while 12% were associated with chronic respiratory diseases and 3% with diabetes.[34] A combination of factors contribute to the rising prevalence of NCDs in low- and middle-income countries, including increasing use of tobacco and illicit drugs, declining levels of physical activity, and changing diets. Limited capacity in low- and middle-income countries to address NCDs, which are mostly preventable, have resulted in higher mortality rates from NCDs than among more affluent countries. In 2008, for example, more than 80% of all NCD deaths occurred among people younger than 60 years in low- and middle-income countries (*Appendix B*).

FY2014 FUNDING

The Administration has requested $9.1 billion to fund global health programs in FY2014, roughly 2% more than FY2012 levels (*Table 1*). Notable increases include a 57% boost for the Global Fund and 13% jump in funding for CDC's global health programs. State-managed bilateral HIV/AIDS programs were the only efforts for which the Administration requested a reduction from FY2012 levels (-10.5%). When compared against the FY2013 Consolidated Appropriations Act, the FY2014 budget request for State-managed global HIV/AIDS efforts was 1.2% lower and the request for the Global Fund was the same.

Table 1. U.S. Government Global Health Funding: FY2011-FY2014 Request (current U.S. $ millions)

	FY2011 Enacted	FY2012 Estimate	FY2013 Request	FY2013 CR[a]	FY2014 Request	FY2012 Estimate -FY2014 Request	FY2013 CR-FY2014 Reque
State Global HIV/AIDS	4,585.8	4,492.9	3,700.0	4,070.5	4,020.0	-10.5%	-1.2%
State Global Fund	748.5	1,300.0	1,650.0	1,650.0	1,650.0	57.1%	0.0%
USAID Global Health	2,498.0	2,625.0	2,504.0	2,641.1	2,645.0	0.8%	0.1%
State-Foreign Operations	*7,832.3*	*8,417.9*	*7,854.0*	*8,361.6*	*8,315.0*	*1.8%*	*-0.6%*
CDC Global Health	340.1	347.6	362.9	n/s[b]	393.0	13.1%	n/s[a]
NIH Global AIDS Research	375.7	392.4	388.9	392.0	399.1	1.7%	1.8%
HHS Global Fund[c]	297.3	0.0	0.0	0.0	0.0	0.0%	n/s[a]
Labor-HHS	*1,013.1*	*740.0*	*751.8*	*n/s[b]*	*792.1*	*7.0%*	*n/s[a]*
DOD Global HIVA/IDS[d]	10.0	8.0	0.0	n/s[a]	n/s	n/s	n/s[a]
Total	*8,855.4*	*9,165.9*	*8,605.8*	*n/sa*	*9,107.1*	*2.1%*	*n/s[a]*

Source: Compiled by CRS from congressional budget justifications, appropriations legislation, and personal communication with OMB.

Notes: Includes global health funding provided through State-Foreign Operations, Labor-HHS, and Defense appropriations.

[a] The FY2013 Consolidated Appropriations act did not specify (n/s) an amount for these programs barring efforts to sum U.S. global health funding (n/a). The amounts listed in this column will likely change due to sequestration.

[b] The FY2014 congressional budget justification did not provide a budget amount for FY2013.

[c] FY2011 was the last fiscal year in which Congress appropriated funds for a U.S. contribution to the Global Fund through Labor-HHS. This category is not applicable (n/a) for all other fiscal years.

[d] The Administration does not typically request funds for DOD global HIV/AIDS programs. Efforts to compare FY2012 funding against FY2013 budgetary requests are not applicable (n/a).

The Administration maintains the proposed budget reductions for some global health activities, particularly HIV/AIDS, reflect increased efficiencies brought about by better integration between programs, greater use of community health workers and nurses, and lower treatment costs. Scaling back funding for bilateral HIV/AIDS programs in some countries, such as South Africa, Kenya, Ethiopia, and also represent efforts to encourage program ownership among countries with growing capacity to manage national HIV/AIDS programs through higher domestic investments, greater availability of resources from other donors, and reductions in HIV prevalence.[35] Despite global HIV/AIDS budget cuts, the Administration projects fulfilling related GHI targets, particularly the target that calls for supporting the provision of HIV/AIDS treatments for 6 million HIV-positive people worldwide by the end of 2013.[36]

GLOBAL HEALTH SPENDING BY OTHER STAKEHOLDERS

The United States provides more official development assistance (ODA) for health than any other country in the Development Assistance Committee (DAC).[37] In 2011, U.S. spending on global health accounted for more than half of all health aid provided by DAC members (*Figure 9*). At the same time, the United States apportions more of its foreign aid to improving global health than most other donor countries. As illustrated in *Figure 9*, Canada is the only other donor that apportions 28% of its ODA to health aid.

Due to varying data collection practices, as described in the section on "Defining U.S. Global Health Assistance and GHI," total amounts reported by OECD on global health aid may differ from national estimates. The Administration reports, for example, that the United States spent $8.85 billion on global health aid in FY2011, while the OECD reports the United States spent $8.33 billion in 2011.

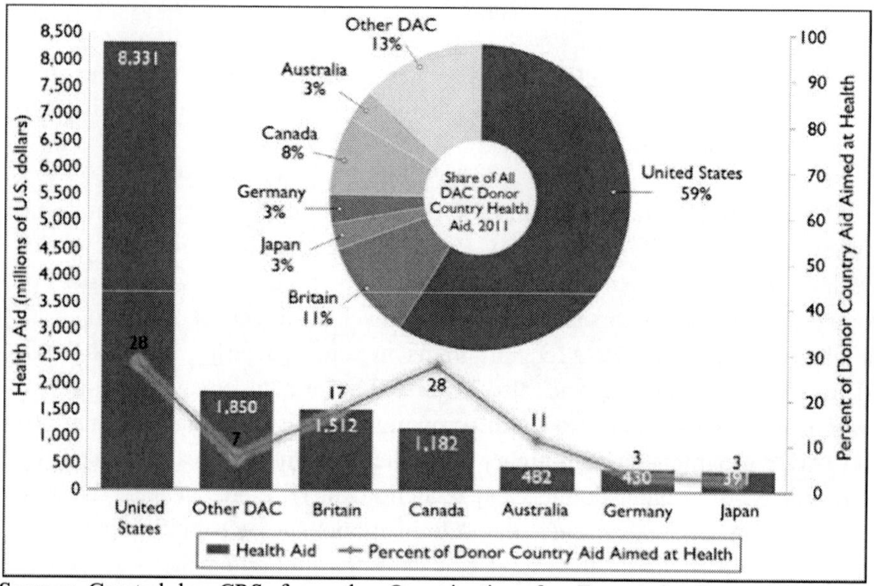

Source: Created by CRS from the Organization for Economic Cooperation and Development (OECD) website on statistics at http://www.oecd.org/statistics/, accessed on February 5, 2012.

Notes: Data in this figure reflects reported spending by DAC members. The data does not include funding from other sources, including European Union institutions, the World Bank or private donors like the Gates Foundation. Health aid levels in this figure include the OECD aid categories of health and population.

Due to varying data collection practices, as described in the section on “Defining U.S. Global Health Assistance and GHI,” total amounts reported by OECD on global health aid may differ from national estimates. The Administration reports, for example, that the United States spent $8.85 billion on global health aid in FY2011, while the OECD reports the United States spent $8.33 billion in 2011.

In 2011, ODA for health by other DAC countries include Greece ($3 million), Portugal ($17 million), Finland ($20 million), New Zealand ($20 million), Luxembourg ($41 million), Switzerland ($67 million), Austria ($74 million), Italy ($91 million), Ireland ($96 million), Denmark ($142 million), Netherlands ($154 million), Korea ($162 million), France ($179 million), Sweden ($182 million), Norway ($183 million), Spain ($200 million), Belgium ($211 million).

Figure 9. Official Development Assistance for Health, by Country, 2011. (current U.S. millions and percent of total).

In 2011, ODA for health by other DAC countries include Greece ($3 million), Portugal ($17 million), Finland ($20 million), New Zealand ($20 million), Luxembourg ($41 million), Switzerland ($67 million), Austria ($74 million), Italy ($91 million), Ireland ($96 million), Denmark ($142 million), Netherlands ($154 million), Korea ($162 million), France ($179 million), Sweden ($182 million), Norway ($183 million), Spain ($200 million), Belgium ($211 million).

The global health funding system is becoming increasingly complicated as a variety of new actors become involved. The private sector and private foundations are playing a growing role in addressing global health. In 2011, for example, spending on global health by the Bill & Melinda Gates Foundation was higher than all DAC countries except the United States. Specifically, the OECD reported that in 2011, the Gates Foundation spent some $2.4 billion on global health, roughly $553 million more than Britain, the second largest DAC donor.[38]

GHI Strategy documents released by the Obama Administration and legislation introduced by the 112th Congress appear to welcome broader engagement in global health, particularly public-private partnerships. There is some debate, however, among global health analysts about how the burgeoning number of players might impact global health effectiveness in general and U.S. influence in this realm in particular. [39] The growth of actors in the global health sector raises several questions:

- How might U.S. influence be affected by the growing number of global health actors, particularly in the area of country ownership?
- How might the United States effectively engage with non-state actors to avoid duplication of resources and improve the sustainability of its investments?
- How might the United States maintain its accountability and transparency standards while reducing reporting burdens?

ISSUES FOR THE 113TH CONGRESS

The U.S. role in global health has been both applauded and criticized. Supporters have celebrated the attention the United States has brought to global health, as well as advancements U.S. programs have helped to make in improving global health. In real terms, donor countries have increased ODA for health since the launch of U.S. global health initiatives like PEPFAR, PMI, and the NTD Program (*Figure 10*). At the same time, some critics have disapproved of the establishment of U.S. health programs that parallel, rather than operate within, national health services, particularly for global HIV/AIDS programs.

Critics contended the U.S programs unnecessarily duplicated national health efforts of host countries and hampered country ownership of health programs.

This section discusses these issues as well as some other pressing global health policy issues facing the 113th Congress.

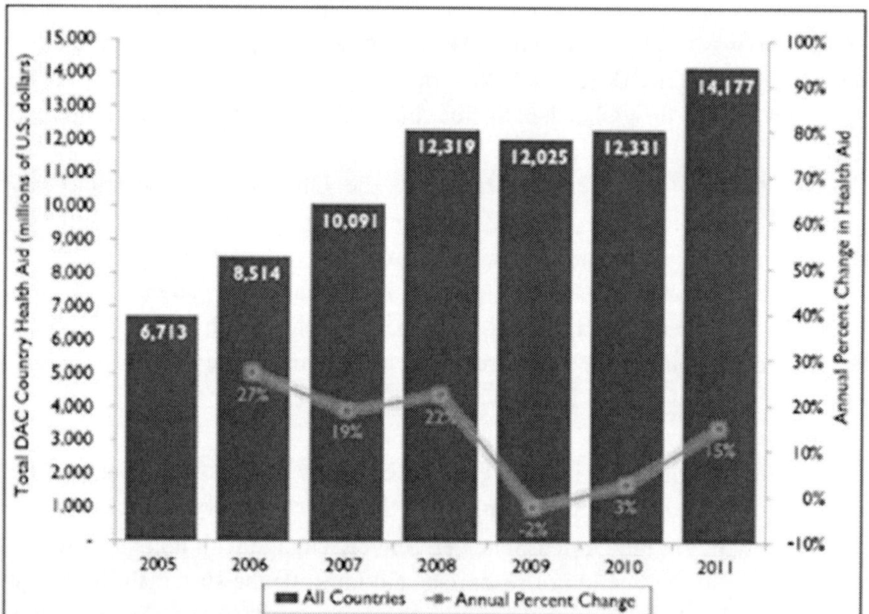

Source: Created by CRS from the Organization for Economic Cooperation and Development (OECD) website on statistics at http://www.oecd.org/statistics/, accessed on February 5, 2012.

Notes: Data in this figure reflects spending by DAC members and does not include funding from other sources, including European Union institutions, the World Bank or private donors like the Gates Foundation.

Health aid levels include the OECD aid categories of health and population.

Figure 10. Official Development Assistance for Health, FY2005-FY2011. (current U.S. $ millions and annual percent change).

Defining U.S. Global Health Assistance and GHI

When President Obama announced the Global Health Initiative, some expressed hope that questions about what programs should be counted towards U.S. global health spending would be resolved. Some believe these questions remain and that some confusion persists about what activities are included under GHI. For example, official documents on GHI spending only cover global health activities funded through PEPFAR and the Global Health Programs account in State-Foreign Operations, even though other agencies and departments outside of State, USAID and CDC play a role in GHI. The Department of Defense, for instance, expends a significant amount of resources on global health,[40] yet GHI documents do not outline the relationship between DOD and the other implementing agencies nor do they explain how agencies like DOD will further the goals of GHI.

Questions also remain about the coordination of global health programs between Washington and the field and whether several long-standing issues with U.S. global health assistance have been addressed, including

- a lack of consensus on what programs to count towards U.S. global health spending;
- an unclear role for each implementing agency in improving global health, particularly through GHI; and
- ambiguous leadership of U.S. global health efforts.

By any calculation, funding for global health has grown considerably since FY2000, particularly through FY2008. Congress has used appropriations and authorizing legislation to direct how those budgetary increases are to be applied and to detail the roles and responsibilities for key global health positions. The Leadership Act, for example, authorized the creation of the Global AIDS Coordinator while the Lantos-Hyde Act authorized the establishment of the Malaria Coordinator. The legislation spelled out the roles of the coordinators, the oversight authority of the positions and the priority areas to be addressed in carrying out related programs.

Congress has not separately authorized GHI. Legislation authorizing the establishment of a Global Health Coordinator could clarify some of the questions regarding GHI, as discussed above. Congress has also not yet considered legislation to authorize the Global Health Diplomacy Office. Authorizing legislation might also be considered as an option for clarifying the role of the GHD office, as well as resolving some of the questions listed in previous sections about the oversight authorities of the office.

Funding GHI

Debates about U.S. global health spending levels are complex and, some argue, distinct from general debates over foreign aid levels because many U.S. global health programs offer immediate life-saving interventions. Several global health advocates argue that U.S. support for global health is critical for scaling up the use of new—and potentially very successful—tools to prevent and treat diseases, including HIV/AIDS and malaria. A number of observers contend that a decline or leveling off of global health spending could threaten U.S. efforts to develop multiyear agreements with governments that call for recipient countries to increasingly assume responsibility over the programs. At the same time, some Members have questioned the impact of U.S. global health investments, criticized corrupt practices by various governments receiving global health assistance, and called for greater commitment to health by recipient countries.[41]

The Administration is reportedly taking steps to address concerns about aid effectiveness and corruption. In 2011, USAID Administrator Rajiv Shah created a suspension and debarment task force to monitor, investigate and respond to suspicious activity.[42] In the same year, USAID released a new evaluation policy that seeks to increase independent evaluation of ongoing projects with results being released within three months of completing the evaluation.[43] In February 2012, President Obama signed an executive order establishing the President's Global Development Council, to be administered by USAID. According to the White House, the council will inform and provide advice to the President and other U.S. officials on U.S. global development policies and practices and solicit input on current and emerging issues in the field.[44]

Maintaining HIV/AIDS Commitments

On World AIDS Day in December 2011, President Obama announced that the United States was committed to supporting treatments for 6 million HIV-positive people by the end of 2013.[45] This announcement followed the May 2011 release of findings, which indicated that early initiation of HIV treatment in discordant couples[46] reduced HIV transmission by 96%. The NIH-funded research found that HIV transmission rates declined precipitously following consistent and proper use of HIV medication due to dramatic reductions in viral loads.[47] The finding was hailed by many as a "game-changer" and led several HIV/AIDS experts to argue that HIV/AIDS could be eliminated as a public health problem.[48] The announcement also led to calls for maintaining U.S. support of HIV treatment around the world.

The United States spends more than any other country on fighting HIV/AIDS worldwide, accounting for 59% of all donor government spending in 2011.[49] Additionally, the United States remains a key donor for multilateral programs, like the Global Fund, accounting for roughly 1/3 of all country donors. Most developing countries are heavily reliant on donors to fund their national HIV/AIDS plans.[50] In Kenya, for example, donors provided more than 80% of the resources needed to support its $709 million HIV/AIDS budget in 2011.[51]

The Lantos-Hyde Act called for the creation of partnership frameworks that would outline plans for increasing country ownership and funding of national HIV/AIDS plans.[52] The U.S.-South Africa Partnership Framework Implementation Plan, for example, envisions reducing PEPFAR aid from the FY2012 level of roughly $484 million to $250 million by FY2017.[53] Similarly, the government of Nigeria, commits to funding half of its national HIV/AIDS program by the end of the framework's five-year implementation.[54]

Most global health experts agree that country ownership of global health programs is important. Some observers are concerned, however, that the United States is hastily drafting partnership frameworks with countries that are not prepared to assume control over national HIV/AIDS programs.[55] The FY2013 budget request, for example, called for a 57% reduction in global health spending for Ethiopia from FY2012 levels. The biggest cut would come from PEPFAR programs, which the Administration proposes decreasing by roughly 80% from $254 million in FY2012 to $54 million in FY2013 (*Figure 11*).

There is some uncertainty about what impact spending cuts may have on national HIV/AIDS plans.[56] In January 2013, for example, global health experts expressed alarm about proposals to drastically reduce PEPFAR funds in Ethiopia. An Ethiopian official reportedly indicated, however, that the government had been expecting the budget cuts and that it will reduce funding for "softer programmatic activities;" employ innovative strategies; and mobilize internal resources to replace the lost funds.[57]

Opponents to sharp budget cuts point to reports and press accounts from South Africa of stock outs, staff shortages, and poor service at several district and national health centers due to poor management of resources.[58] HIV/AIDS advocates are concerned that by shifting HIV/AIDS service to local health centers, patients may not be able to access their medicines in a timely fashion (raising the risk of drug resistance) or may avoid the centers altogether due to the poor conditions.[59]

(millions of U.S. current dollars)

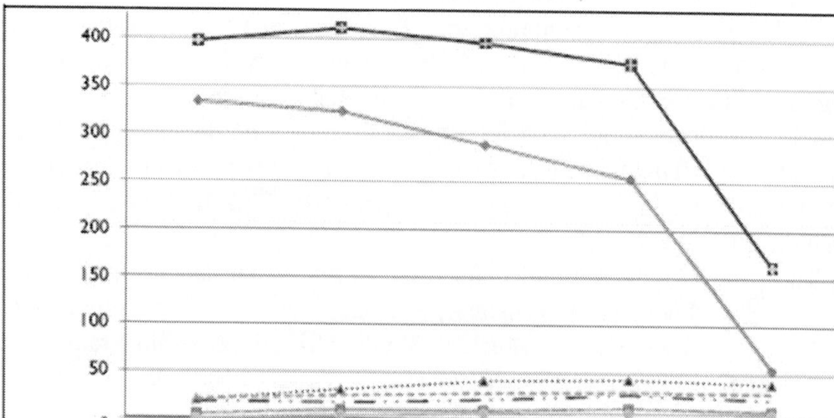

	FY2009 Actual	FY2010 Actual	FY2011 Actual	FY2012 Estimate	FY2013 Request
HIV/AIDS	334	324	289	254	54
TB	5	10	10	13	10
Malaria	20	31	41	43	39
MCH	18	18	21	27	22
FP/RH	21	25	28	30	29
Nutrition	0	4	7	7	7
Total GHI	397	411	396	375	161

Source: Created by CRS from http://www.foreignassistance.gov.

Notes: FY2009-FY2011 actual, FY2012 estimate, FY2013 request. Congress had not yet specified funds for nutrition programs in FY2009.

Figure 11. GHI Spending in Ethiopia, FY2009-FY201.

Reductions of U.S. global HIV/AIDS budgets are distressing for those concerned about taking advantage of recent scientific developments and about maintaining funding for HIV/AIDS treatment programs. This issue is sensitive, since people without medicine will inevitably die. The Administration maintains that reductions in operating costs and increased efficiencies will enable the United States to reach its treatment goals while reducing spending.[60] There is some concern that abrupt reductions in global HIV/AIDS funding will imperil the gains made over the last decade from unprecedented spending levels. Other observers question whether the United

States should vow to continuously increase the number of patients receiving treatment considering HIV-positive people need to be treated for a lifetime.[61]

Extending PEPFAR Authorization Legislation

Funds to carry out PEPFAR have been authorized under two successive authorization acts: the Leadership Act of 2003 (P.L. 108-25) and the Lantos-Hyde Act of 2008 (P.L. 110-293). The acts authorized the appropriation of $15 billion and $48 billion, respectively, for fighting HIV/AIDS, TB, and malaria. Authorization for funds to carry out PEPFAR is set to expire at the end of FY2013. The U.S. Congress has become more divided over issues related to foreign aid in general since Lantos-Hyde was enacted. It is uncertain whether these issues will be sufficiently resolved as to enable reauthorization in the 113th Congress. If Congress does not enact a second reauthorization, PEPFAR activities could continue to be funded through annual appropriations, but Congress might consider whether its priorities could be sufficiently delineated through appropriations alone.

Balancing Bilateral and Multilateral Activities

The appropriate balance between bilateral and multilateral assistance is a frequent point of contention among U.S. policymakers. This debate has intensified in recent years as the Obama Administration has taken several steps to heighten support for multilateral organizations, particularly the Global Fund. The United States is a leading contributor to several other multilateral health organizations, including UNAIDS, WHO, the International AIDS Vaccine Initiative (IAVI), and the GAVI Alliance, among others. Nonetheless, discussions about the appropriate mix of multilateral and bilateral funding have primarily focused on U.S. support for the Global Fund.

Proponents of strong bilateral funding argue that direct U.S. global health spending carries a number of advantages, including the ability to

- strategically direct where and how aid is used,
- more easily monitor and evaluate use of aid and program impact, and
- more rapidly adjust how funds are spent.

On the other hand, some observers maintain U.S. participation in multilateral responses to global health offers distinct advantages, including the ability to

- pool and leverage limited resources, which can capitalize on efficiencies,
- coordinate assistance with a range of donors, and
- provide aid that better aligns with the priorities of the recipient countries.

The debate about the appropriate funding levels for bilateral and multilateral funding can distract from another important issue: alignment of bilateral and multilateral programs. According to a report by WHO, 20% to 40% of health spending is wasted through inefficiency.[62] The report identified several areas in which donors could eliminate waste, namely through aligning financial, reporting, and monitoring practices. By harmonizing the auditing, monitoring, and evaluation of bilateral and multilateral programs, WHO asserted, health staff could use some of the time spent on compiling reports to addressing other health issues.

Supporters of donor harmonization call on the Obama Administration to sign the *International Health Partnership Compact*, an international agreement drafted by the International Health Partnership (IHP+) that calls for the international community to work together to improve the efficiency of health aid.[63] The compact specifically calls on

- *international organizations and bilateral donors* to use national health plans as the basis for funding and planning health aid, ensure efforts to address particular diseases are funded and implemented as part of a broader effort to improve health systems, and be accountable for health aid by annually evaluating, monitoring, and reporting on results;
- *governments* to use national health plans to guide development of health systems, work with all stakeholders (including civil society and international organizations) and ensure that budgets reflect common vision for the health sector, tackle misappropriation of funds, strengthen health and financial management systems, and be accountable to the citizenry and funders through reports on results; and

- *other donors* to use their resources to advance coordinated multilateral approaches to strengthening health systems, continue to invest in learning and evaluation mechanisms to identify best practices, and be accountable and hold organizations receiving support accountable for measuring impact and directing funding to proven successes.

As of May 2013, 58 countries, multilateral organizations, and other donors have signed the International Health Partnership Compact.[64] While the Obama Administration has indicated support for the agreement,[65] the United States has not signed it.

CONCLUSION

Global health has been a central issue in congressional debates over foreign assistance programs and funding levels. Some expect that global health will be an area of ongoing congressional interest, both as a way to potentially reduce overall spending and to improve the effectiveness of aid. In determining funding levels for global health programs, Congress may consider

- ways that the United States can encourage country ownership of global health programs;
- the appropriate balance of funding between bilateral and multilateral programs;
- the role that the United States plays in global health, particularly in relation to other donors; and
- the extent to which the United States can invest in new global health areas.

The rising global prevalence of non-communicable diseases can threaten U.S. efforts to transfer ownership of U.S. global health programs to recipient countries. Many middle-income countries like South Africa face dual epidemics of diseases associated with growing prosperity (diabetes) and persistent poverty (vaccine preventable deaths). In the absence of higher spending levels, bolstering health systems will likely gain greater importance in U.S. global health programs. Such efforts could help countries formulate sustainable plans to address these mostly preventable diseases while addressing infectious diseases that have threatened poor countries for decades.

Along with debating issues related to U.S. global health assistance, Congress may also consider its own role in U.S. global health aid. Congress has exercised growing involvement in shaping global health programs by authorizing the creation of key global health positions, enacting legislation that included spending directives and described congressional priorities. Global health analysts have debated whether Congress's elevated role has helped or hindered the efficacy of global health programs. For example, some argue that congressional spending directives have limited the ability of country teams to tailor programs to in-country needs. Others argue that congressional mandates and recommendations have protected critical areas in need of support and facilitated the implementation of a cohesive global health strategy across agencies.

APPENDIX A. GHI FRAMEWORK

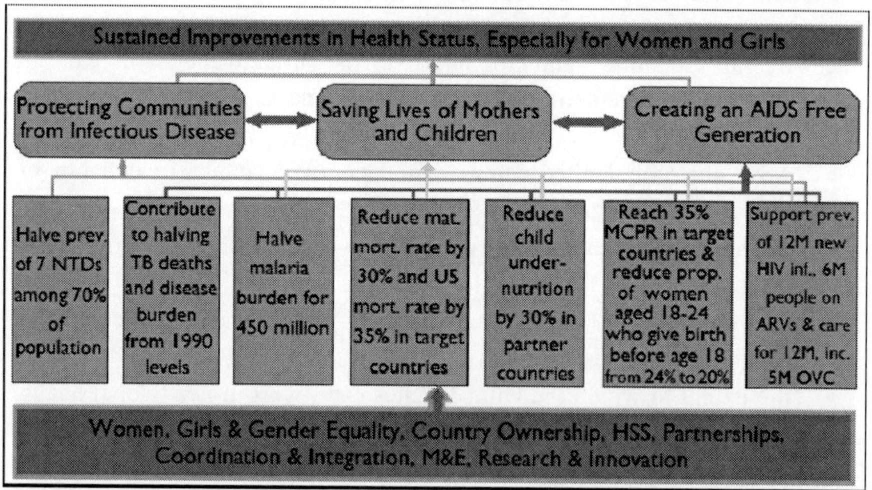

Source: Reproduced by CRS from GHI website, http://www.ghi.gov/about/goals/index.htm, accessed on January 9, 2013.

Abbreviations and Acronyms: anti-retroviral treatments (ARVs), health system strengthening (HSS), maternal (mat.), million (M), modern contraceptive prevalence rate (MCPR), monitoring and evaluation (ME), mortality (mort.), neglected tropical diseases (NTDs), proportion (prop.), tuberculosis (TB).

Figure A-1. GHI Framework.

Appendix B. Non-Communicable Disease (NCD) Deaths Among People Under 60 Years, by Country Income-Group

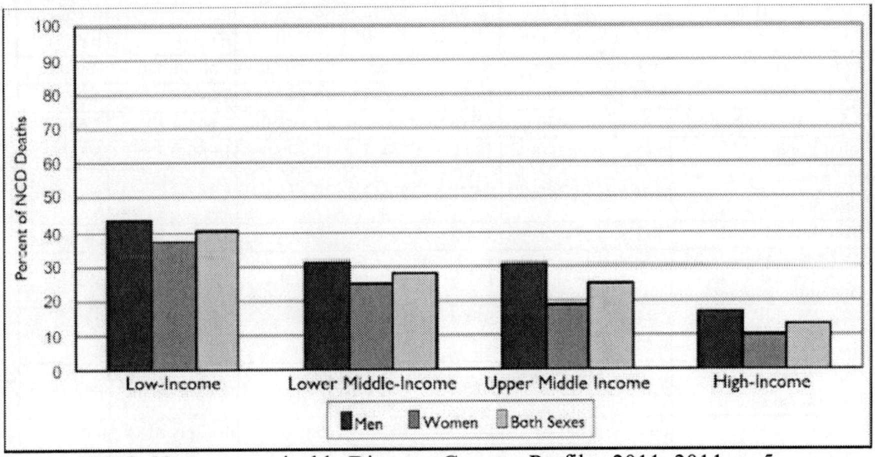

Source: WHO, Noncommunicable Diseases Country Profiles 2011, 2011, p. 5.

Figure B-1. Global NCD Mortality Among People Under 60 Years.

Appendix C. U.S. Global Health Funding, FY2001-FY2014

Table C-1. U.S. Global Health Spending, by Agency, FY2001-FY2014 (current U.S. $ millions)

Agency/Department	FY2001 Actual	FY2002 Actual	FY2003 Actual	FY2004 Actual	FY2005 Actual	FY2006 Actual	FY2007 Actual
State HIV/AIDS	0.0	0.0	0.0	488.1	1,373.9	1,777.1	2.869.0
USAID Global Health	1,115.1	1,297.5	1,572.0	1,451.4	1,314.6	1,456.9	1,653.9
Global Fund	100.0	50.0	248.4	397.6	248.0	445.5	625.0
State-Foreign Operations	*1,215.1*	*1,347.5*	*1,820.4*	*2,337.1*	*2,936.5*	*3,679.5*	*5,147.9*
CDC Global Health	224.1	315.5	344.0	427.9	302.1	311.7	307.6
NIH Global AIDS Research	160.1	218.2	278.5	317.2	369.5	373.0	361.7
Global Fund	0	125.0	99.0	149.0	99.2	99.0	99.0
DOL HIV/AIDS	10.0	10.0	9.9	2.0	0.0	0.0	0.0
Labor-HHS Appropriations	*390.8*	*665.3*	*728.0*	*903.9*	*772.7*	*783.7*	*768.3*

Table C-1. (Continued)

Agency/Department	FY2001 Actual	FY2002 Actual	FY2003 Actual	FY2004 Actual	FY2005 Actual	FY2006 Actual	FY2007 Actual
DOD HIV/AIDS	10.0	14.0	7.0	4.3	7.5	5.2	0.0
Total Global Health	1,715.9	2,076.8	2,803.8	3,642.9	3,964.7	4,715.9	6,163.7
	FY2008	FY2009	FY2010	FY2011	FY2012	FY2013	FY2014
Agency/Department	Actual	Actual	Actual	Actual	Estimate	Consolidated[a]	Request
State HIV/AIDS	4,116.4	4,559.0	4,609.0	4,585.8	4,242.9	4,070.5	4,020.0
USAID Global Health	1,834.2	2,030.0	2,518.6	2,498.0	2,625.0	2,641.1	2,645.0
Global Fund	545.5	700.0	750.0	748.5	1,300.0	1,650.0	1,650.0
State-Foreign Operations	*6,496.1*	*7,289.0*	*7,877.6*	*7,832.3*	*8,417.9*	*8,361.6*	*8,315.0*
CDC Global Health	302.3	319.1	334.8	330.2	347.6	not specified[a]	393.0
NIH Global AIDS Research	411.7	451.7	485.6	375.7	392.4	392.0	399.1
Global Fund	294.8	300.0	300.0	297.3	0.0	0.0	0.0
DOL HIV/AIDS	0.0	0.0	0.0	0.0	0.0	0.0	0.0
Labor-HHS Appropriations	*1,008.8*	*1,060.5*	*1,132.3*	*1,013.1*	*740.0*	not specified[a]	*792.1*
DOD HIV/AIDS	8.0	8.0	8.0	10.0	8.0	not specified[a]	0.0
Total Global Health	7,512.9	8,457.5	9,017.9	8,855.4	9,165.9	not specified[a]	9,107.1

Source: Appropriations legislation, congressional budget justifications, and personal communication with OMB.

Notes: This table does not include funding for the UN Children's Fund (UNICEF), which was appropriated to the Child Survival and Health account prior to FY2004.

Figures in FY2001-2008 include funds appropriated to multiple accounts within State-Foreign Operations. Figures in FY2009- FY2013 only include appropriations to the Global Health Programs Account.

[a] The FY2013 Consolidated Act did not specify an amount.

Table C-2. State-Foreign Operations Appropriations, FY2001-2014 (current U.S. $ millions)

Agency/Program	FY2001 Actual[a]	FY2002 Actual[a]	FY2003 Actual[a]	FY2004 Actual[a]	FY2005 Actual[a]	FY2006 Actual[a]	FY2007 Actual[a]
HIV/AIDS	305.0	395.0	587.7	513.5	347.2	346.5	325.0
Tuberculosis	50.0	60.0	64.2	74.7	79.4	81.8	80.8
Malaria	55.0	65.0	64,6	79.6	79.4	98.9	248.0
USAID Global Fund	100.0	50.0	248.4	397.6	248.0	247.5	247.5
Maternal/Child Health	295.3	315.0	411.9	328.1	347.5	369.6	392.6
Nutrition [c]	n/a	n/a	n/a	n/a	n/a	n/a	n/a
Vulnerable Children	14.9	25.0	26.8	27.8	24.5	12.6	6.5
Family Planning/Reproductive	376.2	402.5	391.0	398.1	396.8	393.5	396.5

Agency/Program	FY2001 Actual[a]	FY2002 Actual[a]	FY2003 Actual[a]	FY2004 Actual[a]	FY2005 Actual[a]	FY2006 Actual[a]	FY2007 Actual[a]
Health							
Neglected Tropical Diseases[d]	n/a	n/a	n/a	n/a	n/a	14.8	14.9
Pandemic Flu/Other	18.7	35.0	25.8	29.6	39.8	139.2	189.6
USAID Total	*1,215.1*	*1,347.5*	*1,820.4*	*1,849.0*	1,562.6	*1,704.4*	*1,901.4*
State Department HIV/AIDS[e]	n/a	n/a	n/a	488.1	1,373.9	1,777.1	2,869.0
State Department Global Fund[f]	n/a	n/a	n/a	n/a	n/a	198.0	377.5
State Department Total	*0.0*	*0.0*	*0.0*	*488.1*	1,373.9	*1,975.1*	*3,246.5*
State-Foreign Operations Total	*1,215.1*	*1,347.5*	*1,820.4*	*2,337.1*	*2,936.5*	*3,679.5*	*5,147.9*
Agency/Program	*FY2008 Actuala*	*FY2009 Actual[b]*	*FY2010 Actual[b]*	*FY2011 Actual[b]*	*FY2012 Estimate[b]*	*FY2013 Consolidated*	*FY2014 Request*
HIV/AIDS	347.2	350.0	350.0	349.3	350.0		330.0
Tuberculosis	148.0	162.5	225.0	224.6	236.0		191.0
Malaria	347.2	382.5	585.0	618.8	650.0		670.0
USAID Global Fund	0.0	100.0	0.0	0.0	0.0		0.0
Maternal/Child Health	449.0	440.1	474.0	548.9	605.6		*680.0*
						not specified[g]	
Nutrition c	n/a	54.9	75.0	89.8	95.0		95.0
Vulnerable Children	14.9	15.0	15.0	15.0	17.5		13.0
Family Planning/Reproductive Health	398.0	455.0	528.6	527.0	523.9		534.0
Neglected Tropical Diseasesd	14.9	25.0	65.0	76.8	89.0		85.0
Pandemic Flu/Other	115.0	145.0	201.0	47.9	58.0		47.0
USAID Total	*1,834.2*	*2,130.0*	*2,518.6*	*2,498.0*	*2,625.0*	*2,641.1*	*2,645.0*
State Department HIV/AIDSe	4,116.4	4,559.0	4,609.0	4,585.8	4,492.9	4,070.5	4,020.0
State Department Global Fundf	545.5	600.0	750.0	748.5	1,300.0	1,650.0	1,650.0
State Department Total	4,661.9	5,159.0	5,359.0	5,334.3	5,792.9	5,720.5	5,670.0
State-Foreign Operations Total	6,496.1	7,289.0	7,877.6	7,832.3	8,417.9	8,361.6	8,315.0

Source: Appropriations legislation, congressional budget justifications, and personal communication with OMB.

Notes: This table does not include funding for the UN Children's Fund (UNICEF), which was appropriated to the Child Survival and Health account prior to FY2004.

[a] Figures in FY2001-2008 include funds appropriated to multiple accounts within State-Foreign Operations.

[b] Figures in FY2009-FY2013 only include appropriations to the Global Health Programs Account.

[c] After the announcement of GHI in 2009, Congress began to appropriate funds for nutrition programs. Until then, nutrition funds were included in appropriations for maternal and child health programs.

[d] USAID received its first appropriation for neglected tropical diseases per language in the FY2006 State Foreign Operations appropriations that directed USAID to make available at least $15 million for fighting seven NTDs.

[e] The Department of State received its first appropriation for managing PEPFAR funds through FY2004 State Foreign Operations appropriations.

[f] Congress provided funds to the State Department for a contribution to the Global Fund for the first time in FY2006 through the FY2006 State Foreign Operations appropriations.

[g] The FY2013 Consolidated Act did not specify an amount.

Table C-3. Labor, HHS Appropriations, FY2001-2014 (in millions of current dollars)

HHS Program	FY2001 Actual	FY2002 Actual	FY2003 Actual	FY2004 Actual	FY2005 Actual	FY2006 Actual	FY2007 Actual
HIV/AIDS	104.5	168.7	182.6	266.9	123.8	122.6	121.0
Immunizations	106.6	133.8	148.8	137.8	144.4	144.3	142.4
Polio	*91.2*	*107.4*	*106.4*	*96.8*	*101.2*	*101.1*	*99.8*
Other Global/Measles	*15.4*	*26.4*	*42.4*	*41.0*	*43.2*	*43.2*	*42.6*
Parasitic Disease/Malaria	n/a	n/a	n/a	n/a	n/a	n/a	n/a
Malaria	13.0	*13.0*	*12.6*	*9.2*	*9.1*	*9.0*	*8.9*
Global Disease Detection	0.0	0.0	0.0	11.6	21.4	32.4	32.0
FE(L)TP/SMDP	n/a	n/a	n/a	2.4	3.4	3.4	3.3
CDC Total	*224.1*	*315.5*	*344.0*	*427.9*	*302.1*	*311.7*	*307.6*
NIH Global AIDS Research	160.1	218.2	278.5	317.2	369.5	373.0	361.7
HHS Global Fund	0.0	125.0	99.0	149.0	99.2	99.0	99.0
DOL	10.0	10.0	9.9	9.9	2.0	0.0	0.0
Labor, HHS, Education Total	394.2	668.7	731.4	904.0	772.8	783.7	768.3
HHS Program	FY2008 Actual	FY2009 Actual	FY2010 Actual	FY2011 Actual	FY2012 Estimate	FY2013 Consolidated	FY2014 Request
Global AIDS Program (GAP)	118.9	118.9	119.0	118.7	117.1		131.9
Immunizations	139.8	143.3	153.7	150.9	160.3		183.0
Polio	*98.0*	*101.5*	*101.8*	*101.6*	*111.3*		*131.0*
Other Global/Measles	*41.8*	*41.8*	*51.9*	*49.3*	*49.0*		*52.0*
Parasitic Disease/Malaria[a]	n/a	n/a	19.8	19.9	19.4		22.2
Malaria	*8.7*	*9.4*	*9.4*	*9.4*	*9.4*		*10.7*
						not specified[b]	

HHS Program	FY2001 Actual	FY2002 Actual	FY2003 Actual	FY2004 Actual	FY2005 Actual	FY2006 Actual	FY2007 Actual
Global Disease Detection	31.4	33.7	44.2	41.9	41.6		45.6
FE(L)TP/SMDP	3.5	13.8	8.5	9.3	9.2		10.3
CDC Total	302.3	319.1	345.2	340.7	347.6		393.0
NIH Global AIDS Research	411.7	451.7	485.6	375.7	392.4		399.1
HHS Global Fund	294.8	300.0	300.0	297.3	0.0		0.0
DOL	0.0	0.0	0.0	0.0	0.0		0.0
Labor, HHS, Education Total	1,008.8	1,070.8	1130.8	1,013.7	740.0	not specified [b]	792.1

Source: Appropriations legislation, congressional budget justifications, and personal communication with OMB.

Acronyms: not applicable (n/a), not specified (n/s), Field Epidemiology Laboratory Training Program (FELTP)/Sustainable Management Development Program (SMDP).

[a] The FY2012 Congressional Budget Justification proposed creating a new funding category, Parasitic Diseases/Malaria, that combined funding for programs aimed at addressing parasitic diseases (like neglected tropical diseases) with those aimed at combating malaria. Since FY2010, CDC operating plans have reported spending in this fashion.

[b] The FY2013 Consolidated Act did not specify an amount.

Table C-4. PEPFAR, FY2001-FY2014 (current U.S. $ millions)

Agency/Department	FY2001 Actual	FY2002 Actual	FY2003 Actual	FY2004 Actual	FY2005 Actual	FY2006 Actual	FY2007 Actual
State HIV/AIDSa	0.0	0.0	0.0	488.1	1,373.9	1,975.1	3,246.5
*State Global Fund*b	*0.0*	*0.0*	*0.0*	*0.0*	*0.0*	*198.0*	*377.5*
USAID Global HIV/AIDS	405.0	445.0	836.1	911.1	595.2	594.0	572.5
USAID Global Fund	*100.0*	*50.0*	*248.4*	*397.6*	*248.0*	*247.5*	*247.5*
State-Foreign Operations	*405.0*	*445.0*	*836.1*	*1,399.2*	*1,969.1*	*2,569.1*	*3,819.0*
CDC Global HIV/AIDS	104.5	168.7	182.6	266.9	123.8	122.6	121.0
NIH Global AIDS Research	160.1	218.2	278.5	317.2	369.5	373.0	361.7
HHS Global Fund	0.0	125.0	99.0	149.0	99.2	99.0	99.0
DOL Global HIV/AIDS	10.0	10.0	9.9	9.9	2.0	0.0	0.0
Labor-HHS Appropriations	*274.6*	*521.9*	*570.0*	*743.3*	*594.5*	*594.6*	*581.7*
DOD Global HIV/AIDS	10.0	14.0	7.0	4.3	7.5	5.2	0.0
Total PEPFAR	689.6	980.9	1,413.1	2,146.5	2,571.1	3,168.9	4,400.7
Total Global Fund	*100.0*	*175.0*	*347.4*	*546.6*	*347.2*	*544.5*	*724.0*

Table C-4. (Continued)

Agency/Department	FY2001 Actual	FY2002 Actual	FY2003 Actual	FY2004 Actual	FY2005 Actual	FY2006 Actual	FY2007 Actual
	FY2008	FY2009	FY2010	FY2011	FY2012	FY2013	FY2014
Agency/Department	Actual	Actual	Actual	Actual	Estimate	Consolidated	Request
State HIV/AIDS[a]	4,661.9	5,159.0	5,359.0	5,334.3	5,542.9	4,070.5	4,020.0
State Global Fund[b]	*545.5*	*600.0*	*750.0*	*748.5*	*1,300.0*	*1,650.0*	*1,650.0*
USAID Global HIV/AIDS	347.2	450.0	350.0	349.3	350.0	not specified[c]	330.0
USAID Global Fund	*0.0*	*100.0*	*0.0*	*0.0*	*0.0*	*0.0*	*0.0*
State-Foreign Operations	*5,009.1*	*5,609.0*	*5,709.0*	*5,683.6*	*5,892.9*	*not specifiedc*	*6,000.0*
CDC Global HIV/AIDS	118.9	118.9	119.0	118.7	117.1	not specified[c]	131.9
NIH Global AIDS Research	411.7	451.7	485.6	375.7	364.7	392.0	399.1
HHS Global Fund	294.8	300.0	300.0	297.3	0.0	0.0	0.0
DOL Global HIV/AIDS	0.0	0.0	0.0	0.0	0.0	0.0	0.0
Labor-HHS Appropriations	*825.4*	*870.6*	*904.6*	*791.7*	*481.6*	not specified[c]	*531.0*
DOD Global HIV/AIDS	8.0	8.0	10.0	10.0	8.0		0.0
Total PEPFAR	5,842.5	6,487.6	6,623.6	6,485.3	6,382.5	not specifiedc	6,531.0
Total Global Fund	*840.3*	*1,000.0*	*1,050.0*	*1,045.8*	*1,300.0*	*1,650.0*	*1,650.0*

Source: Appropriations legislation, congressional budget justifications, and personal communication with OMB. Notes: Rows that are indented and italicized are included within totals of the preceding rows.

[a] The Department of State received its first appropriation for managing PEPFAR funds through FY2004 State Foreign Operations appropriations.

[b] Congress provided funds to the State Department for a contribution to the Global Fund for the first time in FY2006 through the FY2006 State Foreign Operations appropriations.

[c] The FY2013 Consolidated Appropriations Act did not specify an amount.

End Notes

[1] The White House, Infectious Diseases, Presidential Decision Directive NSTC-7, June 12, 1996.

[2] For more on the LIFE Initiative, see CRS Report RL33771, Trends in U.S. Global AIDS Spending: FY2000-FY2008.

[3] For more on PMI and the NTD Program, see CRS Report R41644, U.S. Response to the Global Threat of Malaria: Basic Facts and CRS Report R41607, Neglected Tropical Diseases: Background, Responses, and Issues for Congress.

[4] See for example, White House, "Statement by the President on Global Health Initiative," press release, May 5, 2009.

[5] See CRS Report R41360, Abortion and Family Planning-Related Provisions in U.S. Foreign Assistance Law and Policy and CRS Report RL33250, International Family Planning Programs: Issues for Congress.

[6] PEPFAR, Working Together for an AIDS-Free Generation: World AIDS Day Results, March 14, 2013.

[7] WHO, Millennium Development Goals, Fact Sheet, Number 290, November 2012.

[8] Personal correspondence with USAID, March 29, 2013.

[9] USAID, The President's Malaria Initiative, Sixth Annual Report to Congress, April 2012, pp. 5 and 9.

[10] GAVI Alliance is a public-private partnership focused on increasing access to immunization for children around the world.

[11] GAVI Alliance, GAVI Alliance Progress Report, 2011, p. 7.

[12] WHO, Millennium Development Goals, Fact Sheet, Number 290, November 2012.

[13] Ibid, p. 72 and USAID webpage on family planning.

[14] For background on USAID's global health programs, see CRS Report RS22913, USAID Global Health Programs: FY2001-FY2012 Request; and http://www.usaid.gov/what-we-do/global-health.

[15] For background on CDC's global health programs, see CRS Report R40239, Centers for Disease Control and Prevention Global Health Programs: FY2001-FY2012 Request; and http://www.cdc.gov/globalhealth/index.html.

[16] GHI, "Global Health Initiative Next Steps - A Joint Message," press release, July 3, 2012.

[17] Department of State, "Strengthening Global Health by Elevating Diplomacy," blog post, December 14, 2012.

[18] For more information on these efforts, see CRS Report RL34639, The Department of Defense Role in Foreign Assistance: Background, Major Issues, and Options for Congress; and Kaiser Family Foundation, The U.S. Department of Defense and Global Health, September 2012.

[19] For more on DOD's HIV/AIDS research, see http://www.hivresearch.org/research.php and for DHAAP, see http://www.med.navy.mil/sites/nhrc/dhapp/Pages/default.aspx.

[20] For more information on PEPFAR, see CRS Report R42776, The President's Emergency Plan for AIDS Relief (PEPFAR): Funding Issues After a Decade of Implementation, FY2004-FY2013.

[21] For more information on PMI, see CRS Report R41644, U.S. Response to the Global Threat of Malaria: Basic Facts, and CRS Report R41802, The Global Challenge of HIV/AIDS, Tuberculosis, and Malaria.

[22] The original 15 PMI countries were Angola, Benin, Ethiopia, Ghana, Kenya, Liberia, Madagascar, Malawi, Mali, Mozambique, Rwanda, Senegal, Tanzania, Uganda and Zambia.

[23] For more information on the NTD Program, see CRS Report R42931, Progress in Combating Neglected Tropical Diseases (NTDs): U.S. and Global Efforts from FY2006 to FY2013.

[24] Section 593, P.L. 109-102, FY2006 Foreign Operations Appropriations. The seven NTDs specified in the legislation are: three soil-transmitted helminthes, schistosomiasis, lymphatic filiariasis, trachoma, and onchocerciasis.

[25] For more information on these goals, see GHI, United States Government Global Health Initiative Strategy, 2011.

[26] Personal communication with OGAC, April 1, 2013.

[27] For a list of the benchmarks, see Appendix 2 in State Department, Quadrennial Diplomacy and Development Review, 2010, pp. 217-219.

[28] GHI, "Global Health Initiative Next Steps - A Joint Message," press release, July 3, 2012. For more information on this office, see the "Department of State" section.

[29] Amanda Glassman, "The Office of Global Health Diplomacy: A Christmas Miracle or Lump of Coal?" December 17, 2012.

[30] Personal communication with OGAC, April 1, 2013.

[31] Hillary Clinton, "1,000 Days: Change a Life, Change the Future," remarks, New York City, September 21, 2010.

[32] For more information on the SUN Movement, see http://scalingupnutrition.org/.

[33] John Hoddinott et al., Copenhagen Consensus 2012 Challenge Paper, March 30, 2012, p. 4. A related report on nutrition concluded that the cost-benefit ratios ranged between $23.8 and $138.6. Ibid, p. 37. Nutrition advocates commonly use this statistic to assert that each dollar invested could yield up to a $139 return.

[34] WHO, Noncommunicable Diseases Country Profiles 2011, 2011, p.5.

[35] Eric Goosby, President's Budget Request Reflects Strong Commitment on Global AIDS, Department of State, February 13, 2012.

[36] State Department, Executive Budget Summary, Function 150 and Other International programs, FY2013, pp. 74-80.

[37] DAC is an organization of 24 countries that focus on development. DAC members are part of the OECD, a group of 34 countries committed to international development.

[38] OECD online database at http://stats.oecd.org/.

[39] See for example, Nicole A. Szlezák et al., "The Global Health System: Actors, Norms, and Expectations in Transition," PLoS Medicine, vol. 7, no. 1 (January 5, 2010), p. e1000183; Robert Black et al., "Accelerating the Health Impact of the Gates Foundation," The Lancet, vol. 373, no. 9675 (May 9, 2009), pp. 1584-1585; Kirstin Matthews and Vivian Ho, "The Grand Impact of the Gates Foundation," European Molecular Biology Organization, vol. 9, no. 5 (2008), pp. 409-412; David Stuckler, Sanjay Basu, and Martin McKee, "Global Health Philanthropy and Institutional Relationships: How Should Conflicts of Interest Be Addressed?," PLoS Medicine, vol. 8, no. 4 (April 12, 2011), p. e1001020.

[40] The Department of Defense supports a wide array of activities that improve global health, especially responses to natural disasters and conflicts. The department also maintains laboratories in several countries that conduct research on tropical diseases. These facilities include the Global Emerging Infections System, the Walter Reed Army Institute of Research, Naval Medical Research Centers, and regional commands, including U.S. Africa Command. For more information on these activities, see U.S. Army Medical Research and Materiel Command, USAMRMC Product Portfolio, June 2007.

[41] Shannon Kowalski, The Human Cost of Misplaced Priorities, Open Society Foundation, Blog, April 5, 2010.

[42] U.S. Congress, Senate Committee on Foreign Relations, Statement by Dr. Rajiv Shah, USAID Administrator, Hearing on International Development Policy Priorities in the FY 2012 Budget, 112th Cong., 1st sess., April 13, 2011.

[43] Ibid. Also see, USAID, Evaluation Policy, January 19, 2011.

[44] The White House, "Fact Sheet: The President's Global Development Council," press release, February 9, 2012.

[45] The White House, "Remarks by the President on World AIDS Day," press release, December 1, 2011.

[46] HIV-serodiscordant couples have one partner who is HIV-positive and another who is HIV-negative.

[47] NIH, National Institute of Allergy and Infectious Diseases, "Treating HIV-infected people with antiretrovirals protects partners from infection: Findings result from NIH-funded international study," press release, May 12, 2011.

[48] "HIV Treatment as Prevention: Breakthrough of the Year, 2011," Science Magazine, Special Issues 2011.

[49] Jennifer Kates et al., Financing the Response to AIDS in Low-and Middle-Income Countries: International Assistance from Donor Governments in 2011, Kaiser Family Foundation, July 2012, p. 2.

[50] Michel Sidibé, Executive Director of UNAIDS, "Partners in Treatment," Remarks at United Nations Industrial Development Organization (UNIDO) Industrial Development Board (IDB) 38th Session, November 24, 2010.

[51] UNAIDS, Together We Will End AIDS, 2012, p. 109.

[52] P.L. 110-293, Section 301. Also see the PEPFAR website on Partnership Frameworks.

[53] Department of State, Partnership Framework Implementation Plan in Support of South Africa's National HIV, STI & TB Response, 2012/13 - 2016/2017, August 2012, p. 33, http://www.pepfar.gov/documents/organization/196651.pdf.

[54] Ambassador Eric Goosby advocated the application of the Partnership Framework in his statement for U.S. Congress, House Committee on Foreign Affairs, PEPFAR: From Emergency to Sustainability and Advances Against HIV/AIDS, 111th Cong., September 29, 2010.

[55] Deirdre Shesgreen, "What Should Country Ownership Really Mean as PEPFAR Moves into Next Phase?" Center for Global Health Policy, May 20, 2010.

[56] Amanda Glassman, "Ethiopia's AIDS Spending Cliff," Center for Global Development, September 11, 2012.

[57] United Nations Office for the Coordination of Humanitarian Affairs, "Ethiopia: Concerns Over HIV/AIDS Funding Cuts," IRIN News, January 9, 2013.

[58] Doctors Without Borders, Emergency Intervention at Mthatha Depot: The Hidden Cost of Inaction, January 2013.

[59] Mishack Mahlangu, "HIV Patients Stranded As PEPFAR Funds Dry Up," Health Systems Trust, January 29, 2013; Doctors Without Borders et al., Emergency Intervention at Mthatha Depot, January 2013.

[60] Eric Goosby, "President's Budget Request Reflects Strong Commitment on Global AIDS," blog.aids.gov, February 13, 2012.

[61] Mead Over, Prevention Failure: The Ballooning Entitlement Burden of U.S. Global AIDS Treatment Spending and What to Do About It, Working Paper 144, April 2008; and Neil Patel, Emergency to Efficiency, Harvard Political Review Online, December 5, 2010.

[62] WHO, Health Systems Financing: The Path to Universal Coverage, World Health Report, 2010, p. vi.

[63] See the IHP+ website at http://www.internationalhealthpartnership.net/en/.

[64] See http://www.internationalhealthpartnership.net/.

[65] See USAID, The United States Government Global Health Initiative Strategy, March 1, 2011, p. 8.

In: United States' Global Health Assistance ISBN: 978-1-62948-387-0
Editors: Kurk B. Weller

Chapter 2

THE PRESIDENT'S EMERGENCY PLAN FOR AIDS RELIEF (PEPFAR): FUNDING ISSUES AFTER A DECADE OF IMPLEMENTATION, FY2004-FY2013*

Tiaji Salaam-Blyther

SUMMARY

The President's Emergency Plan for AIDS Relief (PEPFAR) is the largest bilateral health initiative in the world. The 2003 pledge of President George W. Bush to spend $15 billion over five years on fighting HIV/AIDS, tuberculosis (TB), and malaria was considered groundbreaking. The initiative challenged the international community to reject claims that large-scale HIV/AIDS treatment plans could not be carried out in low-resource settings. In December 2002, one month before PEPFAR was announced, only 50,000 people of the estimated 4 million requiring antiretroviral (ARV) medicines in sub-Saharan Africa were receiving treatment. By the end of FY2004, 155,000 people were receiving treatment through PEPFAR.

* This is an edited, reformatted and augmented version of a Congressional Research Service publication, CRS Report for Congress R42776, prepared for Members and Committees of Congress, from www.crs.gov, dated October 10, 2012.

As of March 2012, PEPFAR has supported

- the provision of anti-retroviral therapy (ART) for more than 4.5 million people (up from 155,000 in 2005);
- testing and counseling for more than 40 million people, including 9.8 million pregnant women;
- prevention of mother-to-child HIV transmission (PMTCT) services for more than 660,000 HIV-positive pregnant women, curbing some 200,000 HIV infections among infants; and
- care and support for more than 13 million people, including more than 4 million orphans and vulnerable children (OVC).

Congress first authorized funds in support of PEPFAR in 2003 through P.L. 108-25, the U.S. Leadership Against HIV/AIDS, Tuberculosis, and Malaria Act (Leadership Act). The $15 billion authorization was to be spent on global HIV/AIDS, TB, and malaria programs from FY2004 through FY2008. Strong bipartisan support for PEPFAR in particular and global health in general led to annual appropriations amounts that exceeded authorized levels. During the first phase of PEPFAR (FY2004-FY2008), the Bush Administration spent $18.1 billion on global HIV/AIDS programs.

As the expiration date of the Leadership Act approached, congress-sional support for PEPFAR remained enthusiastic. Members debated a range of issues, but ultimately authorized an extension of PEPFAR. The Tom Lantos and Henry J. Hyde United States Global Leadership Against HIV/AIDS, Tuberculosis, and Malaria Reauthorization Act of 2008 (P.L. 110-293, Lantos-Hyde Act) authorized $48 billion to be appropriated from FY2009 through FY2013 for combating the three diseases. From FY2009 through FY2012, the Obama Administration obligated nearly $26 billion on global HIV/AIDS programs.

As the September 30, 2013, expiration date for the authorization of the Lantos-Hyde Act approaches, it is unclear whether Congress will again authorize multiyear funding for PEPFAR. Bipartisan support for PEPFAR remains strong; nonetheless, congressional debate about key elements of the program has raised some concerns. For example, some Members question the extent to which family planning programs are integrated into global HIV/AIDS activities. At the same time, growing unease about the federal budget deficit minimizes the likelihood that past trends of ever-increasing appropriations for global HIV/AIDS programs will be sustained.

Fiscal pressures may have influenced funding amounts that fluctuated (but mostly remained level) throughout the Obama Administration, a departure from the steady growth in spending seen during the Bush Administration. Financial constraints in the global economy have resulted in similar outcomes during the Obama Admini-stration. Whereas many international donors consistently increased their pledges for fighting global HIV/AIDS throughout the Bush Administration, resources made available by key contributors (such as European nations and the Global Fund) began to stagnate and in some cases declined during the past few years. While contributions by traditional donors have mostly stabilized, Brazil, Russia, India, China, and South Africa (BRICS) are playing a greater role in international HIV/AIDS assistance and are transforming from recipient countries into donor nations. At the same time, some aid recipient countries are increasing investments in their own national HIV/AIDS plans.

This report outlines U.S. spending on global HIV/AIDS programs since the inception of PEPFAR, analyzes global HIV/AIDS funding by other donors, and highlights key issues pertaining to funding that will face the 113th Congress as it considers the future of PEPFAR, including

- whether to reauthorize funding for PEPFAR following the expiration of the Lantos-Hyde Act in FY2013;
- engagement with emerging economies and other non-traditional donors who are increasing their participation in the global fight against HIV/AIDS;
- the impact of U.S. efforts to transition ownership of national HIV/AIDS plans to recipient countries;
- the appropriate funding level for the Global Fund;
- whether to support innovative fund-raising approaches for global HIV/AIDS programs, such as taxes on financial transactions and income; and
- developments that might increase HIV/AIDS treatment costs, including intellectual property rights and drug resistance.

INTRODUCTION

In January 2003, former President George W. Bush proposed that the United States spend $15 billion over the next five fiscal years to fight three diseases worldwide—malaria, tuberculosis (TB), and HIV/AIDS—through the President's Emergency Plan for AIDS Relief (PEPFAR). The plan included $10 billion for programs to combat HIV/AIDS in 15 focus countries; $4 billion for bilateral HIV/AIDS activities in some 100 non-focus countries, global HIV/AIDS research, and international TB projects; and $1 billion for the multilateral Global Fund to Fight AIDS, Tuberculosis, and Malaria (Global Fund).[1] In May 2003, Congress authorized $15 billion in support of the initiative through P.L. 108-25, the U.S. Leadership Against HIV/AIDS, Tuberculosis, and Malaria Act (the Leadership Act).

Congress reauthorized the plan through P.L. 110-293, the Tom Lantos and Henry J. Hyde United States Global Leadership Against HIV/AIDS, Tuberculosis, and Malaria Reauthorization Act of 2008 (the Lantos-Hyde Act). The act authorized $48 billion to be spent from FY2009 through FY2013 on fighting the three diseases; including $5 billion for international malaria programs, $4 billion for global TB efforts, and $2 billion for a contribution to the Global Fund in FY2009.

The Leadership Act and subsequent appropriations were considered groundbreaking. Congress had never authorized or appropriated such sums of funds for a global health endeavor. In the five years prior to the launch of PEPFAR, Congress appropriated approximately $3.1 billion for global HIV/AIDS programs.[2]

In the first phase of PEPFAR (FY2004-FY2008), the United States spent more than $18 billion on global HIV/AIDS initiatives, including the Global Fund. From FY2009 through FY2012, U.S. spending on international HIV/AIDS assistance reached nearly $26 billion. Since PEPFAR was launched, Congress has consistently provided more than the Administration requested for global HIV/AIDS programs (*Figure 1*).

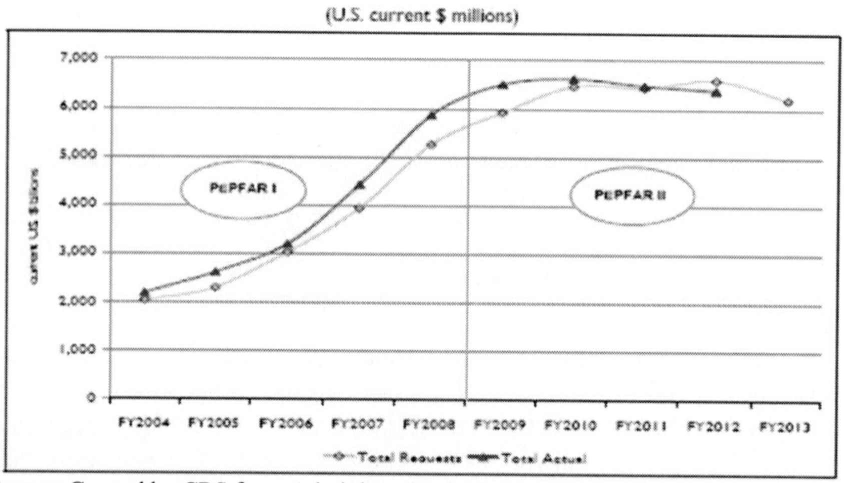

Source: Created by CRS from Administration budget requests and communication with Adam Ross, Global Health Specialist, Office of Management and Budget.

Notes: Includes supplemental funds as well as spending on the Global Fund but not on bilateral malaria and tuberculosis programs. FY2012 funds are estimates.

Figure 1. U.S. Global HIV/AIDS Funding, FY2004-FY2013.

Unless otherwise specified, references throughout this report to U.S. spending on global HIV/AIDS programs include contributions to the Global Fund. It is important to note, however, that U.S. contributions to the Global Fund support grants aimed at fighting HIV/AIDS, TB, and malaria. Donors contributions to the Global Fund can not be directed at any particular disease.

In the first authorization cycle, spending on global HIV/AIDS programs and the Global Fund exceeded the President's proposal by roughly $1.7 billion (*Figure 1and Table 1*). By the second phase, however, the trend reversed: requests outpaced spending levels, which no longer increased annually (*Figure 2*). In FY2011 and FY2012, actual spending on global HIV/AIDS programs was less than the previous fiscal year. It remains to be seen how much Congress will make available in FY2013. Many HIV/AIDS advocates hope larger debates about foreign aid and the federal deficit will not negatively affect PEPFAR funding in the 113th Congress.

U.S. Contributions to the Global Fund

During the second phase of PEPFAR (FY2009-FY2013), Congress continued to debate the role of the Global Fund. Some observers are particularly concerned about the growing share of global HIV/AIDS resources allocated to the Global Fund (*Figure 3*). Although bilateral HIV/AIDS funding has consistently exceeded Global Fund levels, skeptics question whether U.S. priorities can be maintained through an ever-deepening commitment to the Global Fund. Critics also point to concerns about mismanagement of Global Fund resources by some grantees. Supporters, on the other hand, assert the Global Fund complements U.S. efforts by leveraging contributions from other donors and is an important partner in the U.S. fight against global HIV/AIDS.[3] Prompted in part by U.S. concerns, the Global Fund is undergoing reforms. The Board approved the reforms at its 27th board meeting on September 2012.[4]

Congressional appropriations for the Global Fund exceeded requested levels during the Bush and Obama Administrations. The gap between requested and actual spending was the most pronounced, however, throughout the Bush Administration. Presidents Bush and Obama had different views on apportioning bilateral and multilateral HIV/AIDS funds. President Bush never requested that more than 10% of global HIV/AIDS funds be spent on the Global Fund, whereas President Obama requested that up to 27% of global HIV/AIDS funds be reserved for the Global Fund (*Figure 4*).

Table 1. Global HIV/AIDS Requests and Funding, FY2004-FY2013 (current U.S. $ millions)

	FY2004 Actual	FY2005 Actual	FY2006 Actual	FY2007 Actual	FY2008 Actual	FY2009 Actual	FY2010 Actual	FY2011 Actual	FY2012 Estimate	FY2013 Request
Bilateral Request	1,835.0	2,095.0	2,729.0	3,642.0	4,958.5	5,419.4	5,563.0	5,739.0	5,599.0	4,536.7
Bilateral Actual	1,643.0	2,263.4	2,653.7	3,699.2	5,027.8	5,503.0	5,574.0	5,439.6	5,083.1	
Global Fund Request	200.0	200.0	300.0	300.0	300.0	500.0	900.0	1,000.0	1,300.0	1,650.0
Global Fund Actual	546.6	347.2	544.5	724.0	840.3	1,000.0	1,050.0	1,045.8	1,300.0	
Total Requests	2,035.0	2,295.0	3,029.0	3,942.0	5,258.5	5,919.4	6,463.0	6,739.0	6,899.0	6,186.7
Total Actual	2,189.6	2,610.6	3,198.2	4,423.2	5,868.1	6,503.0	6,624.0	6,485.4	6,383.1	

Sources: Compiled by CRS from Administration budget requests and communication with Adam Ross, Global Health Specialist, Office of Management and Budget (OMB).

Note: Does not include funding for bilateral malaria and tuberculosis programs.

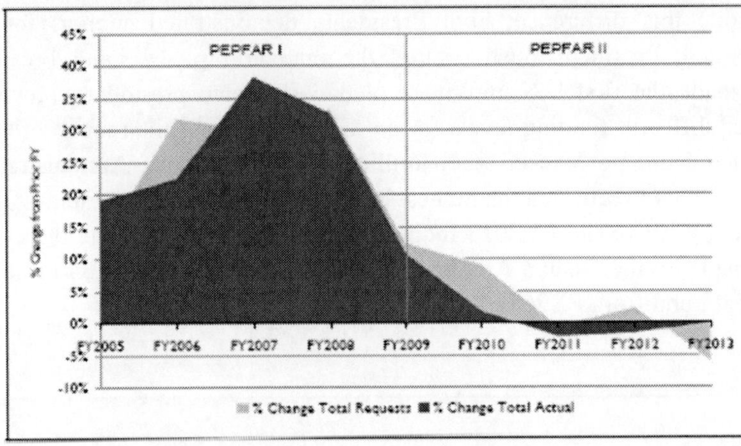

Source: Created by CRS from Administration budget requests and communication with Adam Ross, Global Health Specialist, Office of Management and Budget.

Notes: Includes funding for the Global Fund but not bilateral malaria and tuberculosis programs. FY2012 funds are estimates and FY2013 funds are requested.

Figure 2.Annual Changes in Global HIV/AIDS Requests and Spending, FY2004-FY2013.

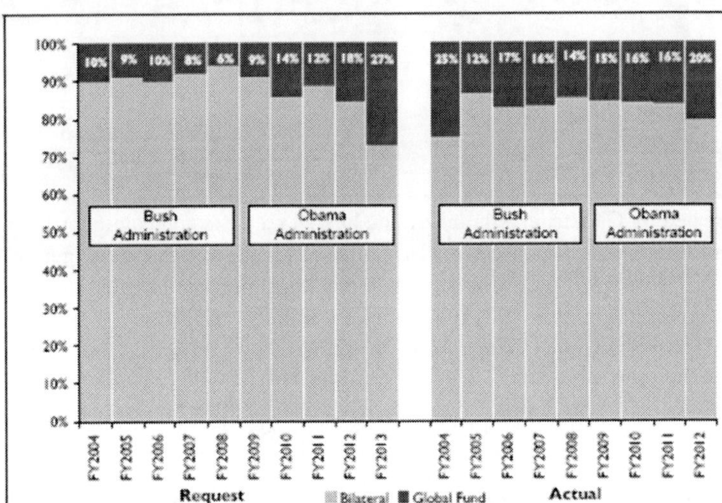

Sources: Created by CRS from Administration budget requests and communication with Adam Ross, Global Health Specialist, Office of Management and Budget.

Notes: Includes supplemental funding, but not spending on bilateral malaria and tuberculosis programs. FY2012 funds are estimates.

Figure 3. Apportionment of HIV/AIDS Resources, FY2004-FY2013.

Despite this difference, both Presidents demonstrated support for the Global Fund. President Bush offered the inaugural pledge, and President Obama made the first U.S. multiyear pledge. The two presidents, however, suggested different funding levels for the Global Fund. While requests for the Global Fund did not exceed $300 million during the Bush Administration, President Obama requested the highest ever pledge to the Global Fund—$1.65 billion in FY2013. The FY2013 request is the final amount of the three-year pledge made by the Obama Administration in 2010 to contribute $4 billion to the Global Fund from FY2011 through FY2013.

(% change by fiscal year)

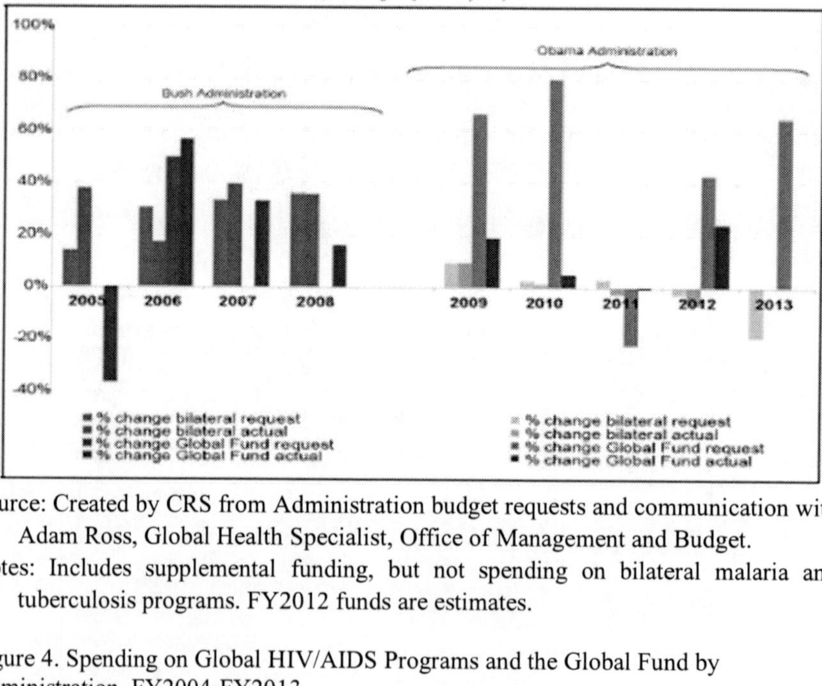

Source: Created by CRS from Administration budget requests and communication with Adam Ross, Global Health Specialist, Office of Management and Budget.

Notes: Includes supplemental funding, but not spending on bilateral malaria and tuberculosis programs. FY2012 funds are estimates.

Figure 4. Spending on Global HIV/AIDS Programs and the Global Fund by Administration, FY2004-FY2013.

EMERGING GLOBAL HIV/AIDS FUNDING TRENDS

Enthusiasm by donors to consistently increase spending on global HIV/AIDS projects has waned, due in part to a weak global economy. Overall spending on HIV/AIDS worldwide, however, has increased. Funding boosts have been driven primarily by budgetary increases among recipient countries.

Between 2010 and 2011, funding from domestic public sources grew by more than 15%.[5] Roughly 41% of that growth occurred in sub-Saharan Africa. Of the estimated $16.9 billion spent on fighting HIV/AIDS worldwide in 2011, roughly half was funded by lower- and middle-income countries (LMIC) and LMIC private entities (*Figure 5)*.

Despite a more austere funding environment, the United States has remained the largest single donor in the world.[6] Of the $16.9 billion spent worldwide on HIV/AIDS in 2011, the United States accounted for 24% of spending from all sources. Among donor countries, the United States provided roughly 60% of all funds for HIV/AIDS assistance contributions. When resources from multilateral organizations are considered, U.S. contributions account for roughly 48% of all foreign aid for HIV/AIDS and 32% of all Global Fund contributions.[7]

(U.S. billions)

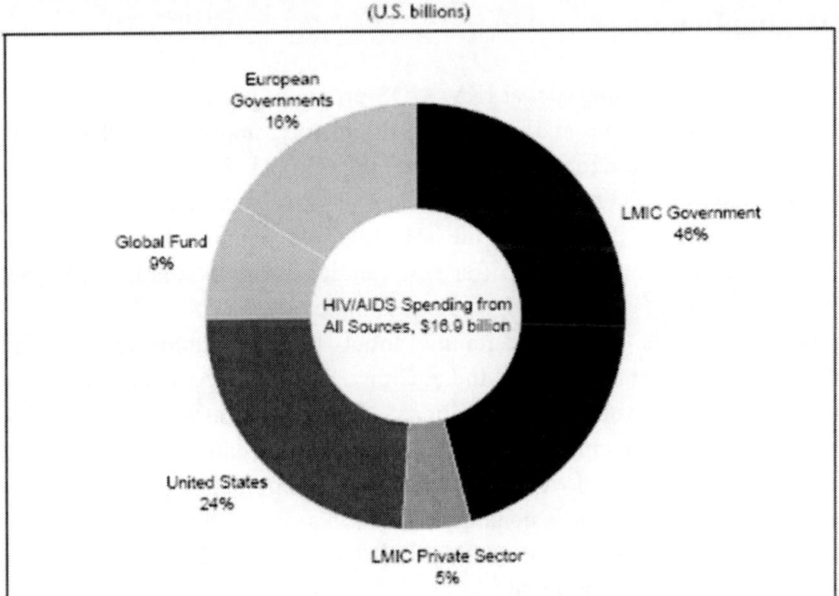

Source: Created by CRS from correspondence with Anja Grujovic, Technical Officer, UNAIDS, September 18, 2012.

Note: Lower- and Middle-Income Countries (LMIC).

Figure 5. Global Spending on HIV/AIDS, All Sources, 2011.

Greater spending by recipient countries on HIV/AIDS in recent years might have been precipitated by congressional mandates for stronger country ownership. In the Lantos-Hyde Act, Congress called for the creation of partnership frameworks to bolster country ownership and enhance the sustainability of U.S. investments.[8] Per the legislation, the frameworks are to outline plans for increasing country ownership of the operation and funding of national HIV/AIDS plans. The U.S.-South Africa Partnership Framework Implementation Plan, for example, envisions gradually reducing PEPFAR aid from the FY2012 level of roughly $484 million to $250 million by FY2017.[9] The framework is based on consistent increases in HIV/AIDS spending by the South African Government (SAG). According to the framework, SAG has raised its national HIV/AIDS budget from $576 million in 2008 to roughly $1.25 billion in 2012.10 As of August 8, 2012, OGAC has signed partnership frameworks with more than 20 countries.

Emerging Donors

Processes for funding global HIV/AIDS programs are changing. Financial contributions from traditional donors are fluctuating, and some global health advocates fear international support for the Global Fund is waning. In November 2011, the Global Fund Board announced that inadequate resources from donors caused it to cancel the scheduled 11th round of funding. The Global Fund does not expect to offer new funding for grants until 2014, after revisions of funding procedures have been completed.[11]

While there is some uncertainty about future funding levels from traditional donors, Brazil, Russia, India, China, and South Africa (BRICS) are playing a greater role in international HIV/AIDS assistance and are transforming from recipient countries into donor nations.[12] Brazil, for example, is helping developing countries manufacture anti-retroviral medicines (ARVs). Russia is donating funds to its neighbors; in 2011, Russia donated $13 million for fighting HIV/AIDS (primarily to border states), and from 2007 to 2010, it contributed $88 million toward AIDS research. India is playing an increasingly important role in offering generic ART to developing countries and is accelerating technology transfer between its pharmaceutical sector and African manufacturers. China is emerging as one of the top five donors for HIV/AIDS research and development (R&D), having provided roughly $18.3 million for research on AIDS vaccines in 2011. South Africa is also increasing its investments in R&D, having spent $10 million on related research in 2011.

At the same time, BRICS have increasingly assumed control over their own national HIV/AIDS programs. Over the past five years, the South African government has boosted its national HIV/AIDS budget fivefold, reaching $1.25 billion in 2012. The Brazilian government has paid for all ART provided through its national programs. India committed to cover at least 90% of all HIV/AIDS expenses related to Phase IV of its National AIDS Control Program (2012-2017). China reportedly paid for roughly 80% of all national HIV/AIDS costs in 2011 after having increased spending on HIV/AIDS programs fourfold from $124 million in 2007 to $530 million in 2011.[13]

ISSUES FOR CONGRESS

The international community has made tremendous advancements in the fight against HIV/AIDS, with the pace accelerating in recent years. In December 2002, one month before PEPFAR was announced, only 50,000 people of the estimated 4 million requiring anti-retroviral (ARV) medicines in sub-Saharan Africa were receiving treatment. By 2011, more than 8 million people living with HIV/AIDS in low- and middle-income countries were receiving antiretroviral treatment, some 20% more than 2010 levels (6.6 million people).[14] Progress has been made as well in preventing mother-to-child transmission of HIV/AIDS. In 2011, approximately 57% of HIV-positive pregnant women in those regions received drugs to prevent HIV transmission; 48% had access to the therapies in 2010.[15]

PEPFAR has played an important role in the global fight against HIV/AIDS. UNAIDS estimates roughly half of all international assistance for combating HIV/AIDS was provided by the United States.[16] Worldwide contributions for countering HIV/AIDS has remained strong even with the global recession and slight declines in HIV/AIDS assistance in 2009 and 2010. Nonetheless, observers question whether global funding for addressing HIV/AIDS will be sustained. Several issues may affect future support for PEPFAR and the global fight against HIV/AIDS, including:

- *PEPFAR Reauthorization.* The PEPFAR program has been authorized under two successive authorization acts: the Leadership Act,[17] P.L. 108-25, and the Lantos-Hyde Act, P.L. 110-293. The acts authorized the provision of $15 billion and $48 billion, respectively, for fighting HIV/AIDS, TB, and malaria. Authorization for PEPFAR is set to expire at the end of FY2013. The U.S. Congress has become more divided over issues related to foreign aid in general since Lantos-Hyde was enacted. At the same time, key elements within the act remain controversial, including those related to family planning.[18] It is uncertain whether these issues will be sufficiently resolved as to enable reauthorization in the 113th Congress. If Congress does not extend authorization of PEPFAR, the program could continue to be funded through annual appropriations, but Congress could lose some of its opportunity to direct how its priorities are implemented.

- *Increased Spending by Emerging Economies.* The Lantos-Hyde Act emphasized country ownership. It is unclear whether U.S. funding levels for global HIV/AIDS programs will continue to rise as the United States and other donors continue to call on recipient countries to increase their contributions to national HIV/AIDS plans. Secretary of State Hillary Clinton has stated at a number of public events that the United States is invested in PEPFAR "for the long haul."[19] Nonetheless, several AIDS advocates are concerned that growing emphasis on transitioning ownership of programs implies declining support for PEPFAR programs. In 2011, fluctuations in donations for global HIV/AIDS were deflected by heightened spending within national coffers. BRICS countries and other emerging economies might also help to increase the global pool of available resources, as well as reduce the pressure on existing donors for fighting HIV/AIDS.
- *Elevated Political Will Among Recipient Countries.* In 2011, the United Nations General Assembly adopted a resolution on HIV/AIDS that, among other things, committed member states to ramp up investments aimed at eliminating HIV/AIDS and work toward closing the estimated $6 billion annual funding gap for combating HIV/AIDS.[20] The declaration called particularly on African countries to allocate at least 15% of their national budgets to the health sector, per the Abuja Declaration and Framework for Action.[21] Some countries, as discussed earlier, have made advancements in this area. Other countries, like Kenya, however, remain heavily reliant upon donors to fund their national HIV/AIDS plans. In 2011, 81% of Kenya's $709 million national AIDS plan was financed by development assistance.[22]
- *Support for the Global Fund.* HIV/AIDS advocates are concerned about the fundraising challenges facing the Global Fund and fear that advancements made through the Global Fund and other donors will be compromised should it scale back operations. The Global Fund

accounts for roughly 18% of spending by donors on HIV/AIDS in low- and middle-income countries.[23] While the Global Fund did not collect sufficient capital to launch a new round of grants in 2012, support from the United States has not abated; it has grown. Since the United States offered the inaugural $200 million pledge for the Global Fund in 2001, U.S. pledges and contributions have increased significantly. In FY2012, Congress appropriated $1.3 billion for the Global Fund and the Administration requested $1.65 billion for the organization in FY2013. Although Congress has continued to increase resources for the Global Fund, it has included language in annual appropriations restricting portions of the contributions, citing concerns about transparency and fiscal malfeasance.[24] Members of Congress continue to debate the appropriate roles of the Global Fund and PEPFAR. This debate is expected to continue in the 113th Congress.

- *Alternative Funding Streams.* Several low-income countries are increasingly considering alternative approaches to financing their national AIDS plans. In January 2000, Zimbabwe launched an AIDS levy that collects a 3% tax on individual and corporate income.[25] In 2011, some $26 million was collected through the AIDS levy, and an additional $30 million is expected to be raised by the end of FY2012. Finances collected through the AIDS levy initiative and from key donors (PEPFAR, Global Fund and the British aid organization Department for International Development [DFID]) is expected to enable Zimbabwe to achieve universal coverage (defined as at least 80% of people in need of treatment) by the end of 2012.[26] Tanzania, Kenya, and Zambia are reportedly considering similar measures. Rwanda and Uganda have also imposed levies to fund national HIV/AIDS plans, but on mobile phone use.[27]

  A non-governmental organization called UNITAID has partnered with several countries to develop innovative mechanisms for funding the global fight against HIV/AIDS. Partnering countries, for example, have agreed to invoke taxes on airline tickets, ranging from $1 for economy tickets to $40 for first-class travel. Roughly 70% of UNITAID's revenues are derived from the air levy for distribution in needy countries.[28] UNITAID and other global health groups also advocate raising funds for global health and HIV/AIDS programs by taxing bonds and derivatives. It estimated that nearly $352 billion (€265 billion) could have been raised in 2010 had G20 nations instituted the levies.[29] H.R. 755, Investing in Our Future Act of 2011, proposes excising a 0.005% levy on currency transactions, in part to fund global health programs, including HIV/AIDS. The bill awaits action by the Committees on Ways and Means and on Foreign Affairs.

- *Cost of Treating HIV/AIDS.* While the world has made tremendous advancements in expanding access to HIV/AIDS, two phenomena may raise the cost of treating HIV-positive people: (1) drug resistance and (2) changes in intellectual property rights. Growing resistance to ART medicine may increase the cost of treating HIV/AIDS as people graduate onto more expensive second-line treatments. In the 2012 UNAIDS report, the organization conceded one of the greatest challenges facing the world is "the inevitably rising costs of drug resistance and the need to provide chronic care for people living with HIV over their lifetimes."[30] Despite these concerns, the World Health Organization (WHO) maintains drug resistance rates remain relatively low in low- and middle-income countries at roughly 6.8%.[31]

The cost of anti-retroviral treatments has fallen tremendously in developing countries over the past decade, from an average annual price of over $10,000 per person to $116 per person for WHO prequalified ART. [32] This decline is a key reason global access to HIV/AIDS treatments has expanded. Indeed, per-patient spending on ART within PEPFAR programs has declined, due in large part to increased use of generic treatments (*Figure A-1).*[33] In FY2009, roughly 90% of all anti-retroviral drugs (ARVs) purchased in PEPFAR programs were generic formulations, up from approximately 15% in 2005.[34] It is important to note, however, that several factors affect U.S. spending on treatment beyond purchase of anti-retroviral treatments, including investments in building renovation and construction, laboratory and clinical equipment and training of ARV providers (*Figure A-2*).

Generic ARVs that are widely used in low-income countries are manufactured primarily in Brazil and India. Some groups, including UNAIDS, are concerned that emergent bilateral and multilateral trade agreements threaten special intellectual property laws that permitted the proliferation of generic ARVs.[35] Of particular concern are developing agreements between the European Union and India that may limit India's capacity to continue producing generic ARVs.[36]

Questions about the pricing of newer, more effective treatments have also prompted some consternation. Members of Congress wrote a letter to the Chairman and Chief Executive Officer of Gilead—a pharmaceutical company that manufacturers ARVs—urging them to consider the impact of elevated ART prices in light of the current economic climate.[37]

APPENDIX. SPENDING ON HIV/AIDS TREATMENT IN PEPFAR PROGRAMS

One of the greatest accomplishments of PEPFAR has been to increase the number of people receiving anti-retroviral (ARV) treatments worldwide, due in large part to increased use of generic formulations. In FY2009, roughly 90% of all ARVs purchased in PEPFAR programs were generics, up from approximately 15% in 2005.[38] Annual per-patient spending in PEPFAR on ART fell from over $1,100 in 2004 to roughly $335 in 2011 (*Figure A-1*).[39]

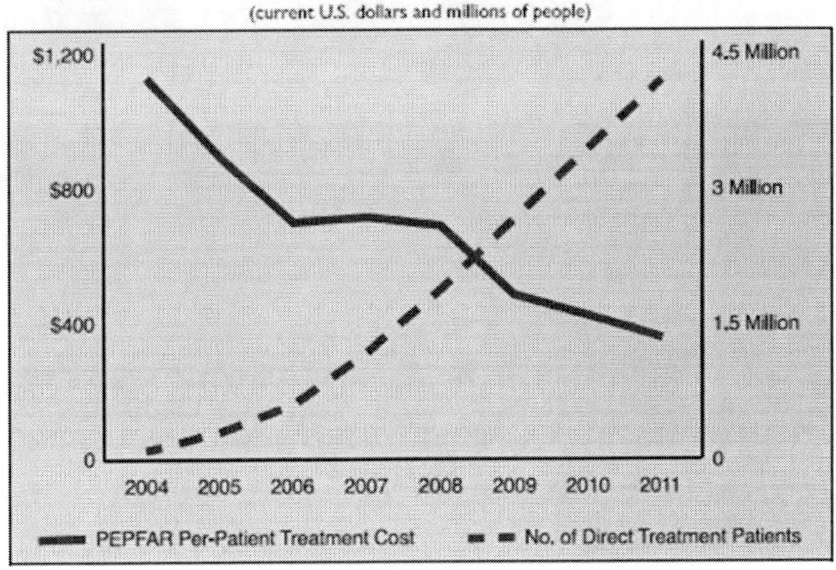

Source: Department of State, PEPFAR Saving Lives Infographic, Fact Sheet, July 2012, http://www.pepfar.gov/documents/organization/195545.pdf.

Figure A-1. PEPFAR Per-Patient Spending on ART, 2004-2011.

It is important to note that spending on anti-retroviral therapy includes a range of activities. The purchase of ARVs comprises roughly 40% of all spending on HIV/AIDS treatment (*Figure A-2).* Non-ARV recurrent costs include clinical staff salaries and benefits; laboratory and clinical supplies; non-ARV drugs for opportunistic infections; building utilities; travel; and contracted services. Investment costs include building renovation and construction; laboratory and clinical equipment; in-service training of ARV providers; and ARV buffer stock to support a reliable supply chain.

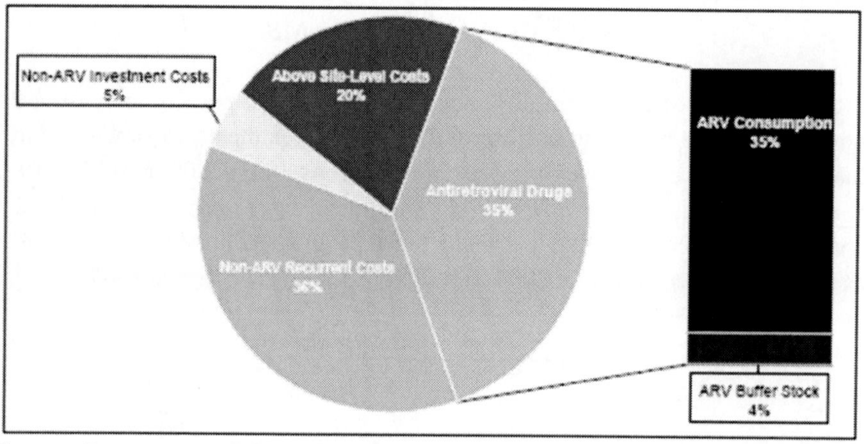

Source: Department of State, Report to Congress on Costs of Treatment in the President's Emergency Plan, July 2010, p. 3.

Figure A-2. ART-Related Expenses, 2010.

End Notes

[1] White House Fact Sheet, "The President's Emergency Plan for AIDS Relief," January 29, 2003, at http://georgewbush-whitehouse.archives.gov/ news/releases/2003/01/20030129-1.html, visited on October 3, 2012. The Global Fund is a multilateral organization based in Geneva, Switzerland, that aims to combat HIV/AIDS, TB, and malaria worldwide.

[2] See CRS Report RL33771, Trends in U.S. Global AIDS Spending: FY2000-FY2008, by Tiaji Salaam-Blyther.

[3] For more information on the Global Fund and congressional discussions about the organization, see CRS Report R41363, The Global Fund to Fight AIDS, Tuberculosis, and Malaria: Issues for Congress and U.S. Contributions from FY2001 to FY2013, by Tiaji Salaam-Blyther.

[4] See Global Fund, Report of the General Manager to the Board, September 13-14, 2012, http:// www.theglobalfund.org/documents/board/27/BM27_02GeneralManager_Report_en/.

[5] UNAIDS, Together We Will End AIDS, 2012, p. 104, http://www.unaids.org/ en/media/ unaids/contentassets/documents/epidemiology/2012/20120718_togetherwewillendaids_en.pdf.

[6] Jennifer Kates et al., Financing the Response to AIDS in Low- and Middle- Income Countries: International Assistance from Donor Governments in 2011, Kaiser Family Foundation and UNAIDS, July 2012, http://www.kff.org/ hivaids/7347.cfm.

[7] Ibid., p. 4, and UNAIDS, Together We Will End AIDS, 2012, p. 10.

[8] P.L. 110-293, Section 301.

[9] Department of State, Partnership Framework Implementation Plan in Support of South Africa's National HIV, STI & TB Response, 2012/13 - 2016/2017, August 2012, p. 33, http://www.pepfar.gov/documents/organization/196651.pdf.

[10] Ibid., p. 9.

[11] Global Fund, Transitional Funding Mechanism (TFM) Information Note, December 12, 2011.

[12] Information in this paragraph was summarized from UNAIDS, Together We Will End AIDS, 2012, pp. 111-112.

[13] UNAIDS, Together We Will End AIDS, 2012, p. 107.

[14] UNAIDS, Together We Will End AIDS, 2012, p. 9.

[15] Ibid.

[16] Ibid., p. 10.

[17] Department of State, The President's Emergency Plan for AIDS Relief: First Annual Report to Congress, 2005, p. 5, http://www.state.gov/documents/organization/43885.pdf.

[18] For more information on the debate surrounding the Lantos-Hyde Act, see CRS Report RL34569, PEPFAR Reauthorization: Key Policy Debates and Changes to U.S. International HIV/AIDS, Tuberculosis, and Malaria Programs and Funding, by Kellie Moss.

[19] UNAIDS, "Secretary Clinton calls for shared responsibility at AIDS 2012," press release, July 23, 2012, http://www.unaids.org/en/resources/presscentre/featurestories/2012/july/ 201 20723aclinton/, and Department of State, Remarks at a Visit to Delft South Clinic and PEPFAR Transition Signing, Cape Town, South Africa, August 8, 2012, http://www. state.gov/secretary/ rm/2012/08/196186.htm.

[20] United Nations, Sixty-Fifth Session, Resolution A/65/L.77, Political Declaration on HIV and AIDS: Intensifying Our Efforts to Eliminate HIV and AIDS, June 10, 2011, http://www. unaids.org/en/media/unaids/contentassets/documents/ document/2011/06/20110610_UN_A-RES-65-277_en.pdf.

[21] For more information on the Abuja Declaration, see http://www.who.int/healthsystems/publications/ abuja_declaration/en/index.html.

[22] UNAIDS, Together We Will End AIDS, 2012, p. 109.

[23] Ibid., p. 110.

[24] For more information on this action and other Global Fund issues, see CRS Report R41363, The Global Fund to Fight AIDS, Tuberculosis, and Malaria: Issues for Congress and U.S. Contributions from FY2001 to FY2013, by Tiaji Salaam-Blyther.

[25] Unless indicated otherwise, information in this paragraph was summarized from UNAIDS, "Zimbabwe: AIDS levy generates new resources for treatment," press release, February 21, 2012, http://www.unaids.org/en/resources/presscentre/featurestories/2012/february/ 201 20221zimbabwe/.

[26] Global Fund, "Global Fund Investments Secure Treatment for an Additional 10,000 People," press release, October 2, 2012, http://www.theglobalfund.org/en/mediacenter/ newsreleases/2012-10-02_Zimbabwe_to_Attain_Universal_Coverage_of_AIDS_ Treatment_by_the_End_of_the_Year/

[27] UNAIDS, Together We Will End AIDS, 2012, p. 107.

[28] See UNITAID website at http://www.unitaid.eu/how/innovative-financing?id=163.

[29] Using $1 = €0.7531 conversion rate. UNITAID, Tax on Financial Transactions, An Implementing Guide, September 2011, p. 11, http://www.unitaid.eu/images/NewWeb/documents/Finance/UTD-Report-TTF_en.pdf.

[30] Ibid., p. 11.

[31] WHO, WHO HIV Drug Resistance Report 2012, 2012, p. 7, http://apps.who.int/iris/bitstream/10665/75183/1/ 9789241503938_eng.pdf.

[32] UNAIDS and UNDP, The Potential Impact of Free Trade Agreements on Public Health, Issue Brief, 2012, http://www.unaids.org/en/media/unaids/contentassets/documents/ unaidspublication/2012/JC2349_Issue_Brief_FreeTrade-Agreements_en.pdf.

[33] See Department of State, Report to Congress by the U.S. Global AIDS Coordinator on the Use of Generic Drugs in the President's Emergency Plan for AIDS Relief, May 2008, http://www.pepfar.gov/documents/organization/ 105842.pdf.

[34] Department of State, Making Smart Investments to Increase Impact and Efficiency and Save More Lives, Fact Sheet, July 2012, http://www.pepfar.gov /documents/organization/ 195478.pdf.

[35] For more information on international intellectual property rights agreements and HIV, see CRS Report RL34292, Intellectual Property Rights and International Trade, by Shayerah Ilias and Ian F. Fergusson.

[36] Patralekha Chatterjee, "India-EU Free-Trade Pact Could Stifle Generics Industry," The Lancet, vol. 377, no. 9774 (April 16, 2011), pp. 1305-1306.

[37] Letter from Alcee Hastings, Member of Congress, et al. to Dr. John C. Martin, Chairman and Chief Executive Officer, Gilead Sciences, Inc., August 1, 2012, http://alceehastings .house.gov/images/stories/PDFs/Rep._Hastings_-_Letter_to_Gilead_-_8.1.12.pdf.

[38] Department of State, Making Smart Investments to Increase Impact and Efficiency and Save More Lives, Fact Sheet, July 2012, http://www.pepfar.gov/documents/organization/ 195478.pdf.

[39] Department of State, The President's Emergency Plan for AIDS Relief Eighth Annual Report to Congress, 2012, p. 3, http://www.pepfar.gov/documents/organization/188019.pdf.

In: United States' Global Health Assistance ISBN: 978-1-62948-387-0
Editors: Kurk B. Weller

Chapter 3

THE GLOBAL FUND TO FIGHT AIDS, TUBERCULOSIS, AND MALARIA: ISSUES FOR CONGRESS AND U.S. CONTRIBUTIONS FROM FY2001 TO FY2013*

Tiaji Salaam-Blyther and Alexandra E. Kendall

SUMMARY

The Global Fund to Fight AIDS, Tuberculosis, and Malaria (Global Fund, or the Fund) was established in 2002 as a public-private partnership that could provide significant financial support for global responses to HIV/AIDS, tuberculosis (TB), and malaria. By the end of 2011, the Global Fund had approved roughly $22.6 billion to help 150 countries fight these three diseases. According to the Global Fund, from 2002 through 2011, it had supported AIDS treatment for 3.3 million HIV-positive people, anti-tuberculosis treatment for 8.6 million people, and 230 million insecticide-treated nets for the prevention of malaria, saving about 7.7 million lives.

In November 2011, the Global Fund Board announced that due to inadequate resources from donors, it would cancel its 11th round of funding, but would maintain support for existing activities to avoid

---

* This is an edited, reformatted and augmented version of a Congressional Research Service publication, CRS Report for Congress R41363, prepared for Members and Committees of Congress, from www.crs.gov, dated May 15, 2012.

disruptions in ongoing services. The Fund also announced that it expected to offer new funding for grants in 2014.

The United States has demonstrated strong support for the Global Fund since making a founding pledge in 2001. U.S. officials have served on several Global Fund boards, U.S. contributions to the Fund have surpassed those of any other country, and U.S. global HIV/AIDS, TB, and malaria programs have been increasingly coordinated with Global Fund activities. Donors last met on October 4, 2010, to make their pledges for the Global Fund over the next three years. There, the United States made its first multiyear pledge to the Fund of $4 billion.

Despite rigorous debate on the overall budget and the role of foreign aid in particular, the 112th Congress has maintained support for the Global Fund. In both FY2011 and FY2012, Congress appropriated $1.05 billion for the Global Fund, excluding rescissions. In order to meet the $4 billion multiyear pledge made in 2010, the President's FY2013 budget request included $1.65 billion for the Global Fund, a significant increase from previous years. As part of the budget request, the Administration requested a transfer of $250 million from the State Department's FY2012 bilateral HIV/AIDS funding to the Global Fund, bringing the estimated FY2012 funding level to $1.3 billion.

Global health advocates urge Congress to meet the President's FY2013 request for the Fund in order to support the sustainability of its activities and to encourage continued contributions from other donors. Although Congress has traditionally been a strong supporter of the Fund, several issues may affect congressional views about the Fund in the future. Such factors include the following:

Fiscal austerity. Proposals to reduce federal spending continue to dominate foreign aid debates, with some Members of Congress aiming to target foreign aid accounts, including those for global health, in an attempt to balance the budget. At the same time, others argue that cutting back on the relatively small size of foreign aid (about 1% of total budget authority) will do little to cut the deficit, but could imperil the lives of millions.

Oversight and transparency. In early 2011, reports about misuse of Global Fund resources in some grants ignited a debate about corruption in foreign aid in general, and in the Global Fund in particular. Some have called for donors to withhold support for the Fund until better safeguards are established. Others argue the Fund should not be penalized for oversight shortcomings, which are familiar to many aid programs.

Role of the Global Fund in U.S. global health policy. When the Global Fund was established, U.S. bilateral investments in HIV/AIDS, malaria, and TB were relatively small. Since then, U.S. bilateral investments in fighting these diseases have grown significantly, particularly since the President's Emergency Plan for AIDS Relief (PEPFAR) and the President's Malaria Initiative (PMI) were launched in 2003 and 2005, respectively. Some observers advocate allocating the majority of U.S. funds for global HIV/AIDS and malaria to bilateral programs to ensure sufficient control and oversight of funds. On the other hand, other analysts argue that the Global Fund represents a more efficient and flexible funding mechanism than bilateral programs and offers the United States the ability to pool funds and share risk with other donors, which some believe is particularly important given the challenges of the current fiscal environment.

This report provides background information on the Global Fund, outlines U.S. funding for the Fund, discusses changes the Global Fund has made to improve the efficiency of its programs and address allegations of corruption, and analyzes issues Congress might consider as it debates the appropriate level of U.S support to provide the Fund.

BACKGROUND

The Global Fund to Fight AIDS, Tuberculosis, and Malaria (Global Fund, or the Fund) was established in January 2002 as a public-private partnership to provide significant financial support for global responses to HIV/AIDS, tuberculosis (TB), and malaria. At that time, health experts and advocates were particularly concerned about the rapid spread of HIV/AIDS around the world, the massive numbers of deaths that resulted from HIV infection, and limited access to treatments against the three diseases, particularly HIV/AIDS. Health specialists also noted that co-infection seemed to hasten the rate at which people succumbed to any of the three diseases. Despite expanded access to care and treatment over the past decade, HIV/AIDS, TB, and malaria continue to be three of the world's leading causes of morbidity and mortality around the world.

The Global Fund was developed to be an innovative financing mechanism that would attract additional financial resources for the global fight against the three diseases in developing countries. It was never intended to directly implement related programs.[1] Several distinguishing characteristics purported to make this new entity a unique one, including

- with no implementation mandate, the Global Fund would have relatively low overhead expenses;
- rigorous monitoring and evaluation requirements could ensure performance-based funding;

- transparency in decision-making, including grant funding, could support accountability; and
- partnerships among governments, the private sector, and civil society would be created and expanded, due in part to the grant development process.

The Fund's Board meets at least twice annually to discuss governance issues, such as grant approval. Nineteen Board seats are rotated among seven donor countries, seven developing countries, and five representatives from civil society and the private sector, including one representative of a non-governmental organization (NGO) from a developing country, one representative of an NGO from a developed country, one representative of the private sector, one representative of a private foundation, and one representative of an NGO who is a person living with HIV/AIDS or from a community living with TB or malaria.[2] The United States holds a permanent Board seat.

In 2001 and 2002, donors pledged $947.2 million to launch the Global Fund. In its first round of considering grants, the Global Fund committed to support 58 programs in 43 countries, amounting to $616 million for the first two years of implementation. In December 2010, the Global Fund Board announced that it would support the 10th round of grant proposals, valued at more than $1.7 billion for the first two years of project implementation. Over five years, the Global Fund could expend some $4.7 billion on these grants if performance requirements are met and resources are available.[3] By the end of 2011, the Global Fund had approved roughly $22.6 billion to help 150 countries fight HIV/AIDS, TB, and malaria. As of mid-February, 2012, almost 70% of all approved funding had been disbursed, amounting to over $15 billion.[4]

Since its establishment, the Global Fund has become one of the world's largest donors supporting HIV/AIDS, TB, and malaria programs in developing countries. In 2009, the Fund accounted for 21% of global spending on HIV/AIDS, 65% of spending on TB in the 22 high-burden countries, and 65% of global malaria funding.[5] The Global Fund estimated that by the end of 2011, the programs it supports had saved over 7.7 million lives. Grants supported by the Global Fund have reportedly provided

- AIDS treatment for 3.3 million HIV-positive people,
- anti-tuberculosis treatment for 8.6 million people, and
- 230 million insecticide-treated nets for the prevention of malaria.[6]

RECENT DEVELOPMENTS

In November 2011, the Global Fund Board announced that due inadequate resources from donors, it would cancel its 11th round of funding. The Global Fund expects to offer new funding for grants in 2014. Until then, in order to avoid any disruptions in ongoing services, the Board has instituted a Transitional Funding Mechanism for programs that

- face disruption of essential services, currently supported by the Global Fund, and
- for which no alternative sources of funding can be secured.[7]

At the November 2011 board meeting, the Global Fund Board adopted a new five-year strategy for 2012-2016, which supports more aggressive management and oversight of grants, encourages more flexibility in tailoring activities to specific country's needs, and embraces more country ownership of programs through increased involvement of country governments (see *Text Box*).[8] The Board also approved the Global Fund's "Consolidated Transformation Plan,"[9] developed to improve Global Fund governance, operations, and fiduciary controls, as recommended by a report released in September 2011 by the High-Level Independent Review Panel on Fiduciary Controls and Oversight Mechanisms of the Global Fund.[10]

In January 2012, the Executive Director of the Global Fund announced his decision to step down. In response, the Global Fund created a new position of General Manager, charged with overseeing the implementation of the Consolidated Transformation Plan.

Highlights of The Global Fund Strategy 2012-2016: Investing for Impact

The 2012-2016 Global Fund strategy outlines how the Global Fund will build on past successes, address new challenges, and better "invest for impact."

The strategy sets new targets of saving 10 million lives and preventing 140 million to180 million new infections from HIV/AIDS, TB, and malaria between 2012 and 2016. To reach these goals, the strategy outlines five strategic objectives:

1) Invest more strategically in areas with high potential for impact and strong value for money, and fund based on countries' national strategies.
2) Evolve the funding model to provide funding in a more proactive, flexible, predictable, and effective way.
3) Actively support grant implementation success through more active grant management and better engagement with partners.
4) Promote and protect human rights in the context of the three diseases.

Sustains the gains, mobilize resources—by increasing the sustainability of supported programs and attracting additional funding from current and new sources.

Global Fund Structure and Performance-Based Funding Process

The Global Fund was established to extend life-saving measures to the world's poorest. In many of these countries, including post-conflict and fragile states, implementing organizations have weak programmatic and oversight capacity. In light of these conditions, the Global Fund developed a performance-based system that has served as a cornerstone of its operations since the effort was launched. The system relies on seven main actors, including the

- *Country Coordinating Mechanism (CCM),* a country-level partnership of stakeholders, responsible for developing and submitting grant proposals, nominating Principal Recipients, and providing oversight to grant implementation.
- *Principal Recipient*, the designated in-country organizations chosen by the CCM to receive funding from the Fund, implement programs, and distribute funds to sub-recipients.
- *Sub-Recipient,* an organization contracted by the Principal Recipient of the grant to assist in implementing program activities.
- *Local Fund Agent,* a contracted entity that provides independent and routine monitoring and financial audits of the Global Fund disbursements and activities.

- *Secretariat,* responsible for day-to-day operations, including mobilizing resources, overseeing grant implementation, providing support to the Board, and reporting on the Fund's activities to the Board and the public.
- *Technical Review Board,* an independent panel of experts in health and development who review eligible grants proposals for technical merit.
- *The Global Fund Board,* responsible for overall governance of the Fund.

Through the performance-based system, the Global Fund has integrated grant oversight at various levels, including

- internal control mechanisms instituted by Principal Recipients;
- independent in-country verification and oversight mechanisms established by Local Fund Agents;
- annual audits of principal and sub-recipients by an external, independent body;
- monitoring of grant implementation by the Secretariat;
- audits and investigations conducted by the Office of the Inspector General; and[11]
- oversight provided by Global Fund Board and its committees.

Upon approving grant proposals, the Global Fund commits to providing sufficient resources to finance the first two years of the program. In order to receive subsequent financing, programs must demonstrate results against performance targets that are spelled out in the grant proposals (*Figure 1*).[12]

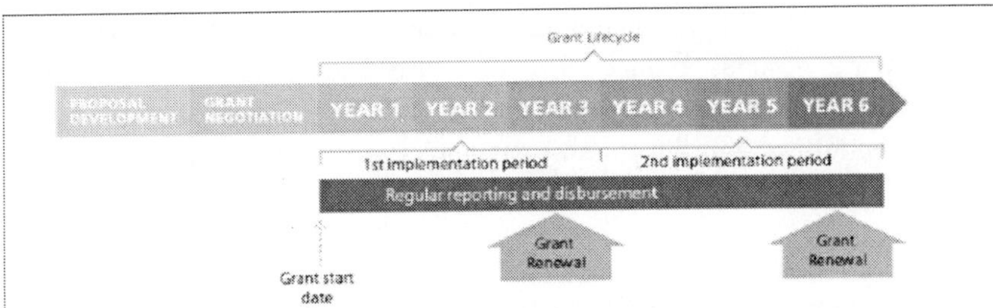

Source: Global Fund, Performance-Based Funding at the Global Fund, http://www.theglobalfund.org/en/ performancebasedfunding/grantlifecycle/, February 2012.

Figure 1. Performance-Based Funding at the Global Fund.

Over the lifetime of a grant, performance-based indicators are developed and monitored in four key stages:

1) *Proposal development.* Applicants develop and submit proposals to the Global Fund Secretariat that include output, outcome and impact indicators, and targets defined by the countries themselves. If the proposal is approved, these form the basis for measuring the performance of a grant.
2) *Grant negotiation.* Upon approval, the Global Fund negotiates the terms of grant agreements, legally binding contracts that clearly indicate time-bound targets to measure the performance of the grants. At this stage, monitoring and evaluation systems are also assessed. The Global Fund recommends that 5%-10% of grant budgets are used for monitoring and evaluation.
3) *Performance-based disbursements.* Over the course of a grant's life cycle, the Principal Recipient reports regularly to the Global Fund on results, expenditures, and any deviations from or corrective actions to program activities. The Local Fund Agent, an independent contractor based in the country, verifies the Principal Recipient's programmatic and financial reports and makes recommendations to the Global Fund on the amount to be disbursed for the next period of implementation. The Secretariat evaluates the overall performance of the grant, assigns a rating, and decides on the next disbursement amount. Lack of progress triggers a request by the Secretariat for corrective action and may also result in reduced disbursements.
4) *Grant renewal.* Toward the end of Phase 1 (first two years of implementation), the Global Fund evaluates each grant to ensure that funding is managed and spent efficiently and programs are achieving expected results. At this point, the Fund decides whether to continue funding grants, reduce funding, direct investments in systems strengthening, or stop funding altogether.[13] Grants demonstrating potential for significant and sustainable impact can receive additional funding for up to six years through the "Rolling Continuation Channel."

Consistent with its performance-based model, the Global Fund reports that it has terminated, suspended, or discontinued grants or replaced principal recipients in cases of uncorrected inadequate performance.

U.S. SUPPORT OF THE GLOBAL FUND

Since the Global Fund was established, the United States has been a strong supporter of the organization. Officials from the Department of State, the United States Agency for International Development (USAID), and the United States Department of Health and Human Services (HHS) were all engaged in the creation of the Global Fund, and former Secretary of HHS Tommy Thompson was later elected as the second Chair of the Global Fund's Board. At present, U.S. officials from various agencies sit on several Global Fund Boards.

The Obama Administration has signaled its intention to maintain that support. In a March 2011 statement[14] and at a House hearing, the U.S. Global AIDS Coordinator, Ambassador Eric Goosby, linked the success of U.S. bilateral HIV/AIDS programs under the President's Emergency Plan for AIDS Relief (PEPFAR) to the continuance of the Global Fund:

> Our dependency on the Global Fund is a real one.... The Global Fund creates a platform and conduit for other countries who do not have bilateral programs to contribute to the care and prevention and treatment dollars for HIV/AIDS as well as TB and malaria.... We plan together and look at how we can converge in any given country to where Global Fund is doing one thing, we're doing something that is complementary or expansive or other than they are doing so our programmatic imprint is amplified in our ability to impact the diseases that both the Global Fund focuses on as well as the HIV/AIDS and TB. Without them, our footprint and impact would diminish.[15]

In the Fund's first budget period, U.S. donations accounted for 33% of all contributions to the Fund, with the United States having provided $300 million of the $894.3 million contributed in the 2001-2002 budget period. Since then, the United States has remained a key contributor to the Fund (*Table 1*). On October 4, 2010, when Global Fund donors met to make 2011-2013 pledges, the United States made its first multiyear pledge to the Fund of $4 billion.

Congress has historically appropriated U.S. contributions to the Global Fund through two appropriations bills: State, Foreign Operations; and Labor, Health and Human Services, and Education. The conference reports (H.Rept. 112-331) accompanying the FY2012 Consolidated Appropriations Act (P.L. 112-74) specified that appropriations for the Global Fund would be funded in whole through Division I (Department of State, Foreign Operations, and

Related Programs). During the Bush Administration, Congress consistently exceeded budgetary requests for the Global Fund and appropriated roughly $3.6 billion for the Fund from FY2001 to FY2008. Congressional support for the Global Fund has continued through the Obama Administration, with appropriations exceeding requested levels each year, except in FY2012 (Table 2).

Despite this support, appropriations for the Global Fund have remained constant since FY2010. In FY2011 and FY2012, appropriations for the Fund remained at $1.05 billion.

Table 1. Total Global Fund Contributions and Pledges(current $ U.S. millions and percentages)

Contributor	Paid as of 01/31/2012	% of Total Paid	Total Pledges as of 01/31/2012	% of Total Pledges
United States	6,079.9	28.0%	9,506.9	31.0%
European Union Countries	9,763.7	44.9%	12,834.8	41.8%
European Commission	1,351.3	6.2%	1,634.1	5.3%
Other Countries	3,528.1	16.2%	5,000.2	16.3%
Non-Governmental Donors	1,010.2	4.6%	1,700.0	5.5%
Total	21,736.7	100.0%	30,676.0	100.0%

Source: Global Fund, Pledges and Contributions, See http://www.theglobalfund.org /en/about/donors/.

In order to meet his multiyear pledge to the Fund, made in 2010, as part of the FY2013 budget request, President Obama requests that the Fund receive an addition $250 million in FY2012 through a transfer of funds from the State Department's bilateral HIV/AIDS funding from that year. Likewise, despite proposing reductions for most bilateral global health programs, the Administration requests $1.65 billion for the Global Fund in FY2013, some 57% higher than FY2012-enacted levels, and 27% higher than FY2012 estimated levels, which take into account the $250 million transfer.

Table 2. U.S. Contributions to the Global Fund, FY2001-FY2013 (current U.S. $ millions)

	FY 2001-FY 2003 Actual	FY 2004 Actual	FY 2005 Actual	FY 2006 Actual	FY 2007 Actual	FY 2008 Actual	FY 2009 Actual	FY 2010 Actual	FY 2011 Actual	FY 2012 Esti-mate	FY2013 Request
Foreign											
Operations	398.4	397.6	248.0	445.5	625.0	545.5	700.0	750.0	748.5	1,300.0	1,650.0
Labor/HHS	224.0	149.1	99.2	99.0	99.0	294.8	300.0	300.0	297.3	0.0	0.0
FY2004											
Carry-over	n/a	(87.8)	87.8	n/a	n/a	n/a	n/a	n/a	n/a	n/a	n/a
Total	622.4	458.9	435.0	544.5	724.0	840.3	1,000.0	1,050.0	1,045.8	1,300.0	1,650.0

Source: CRS analysis of appropriations legislation and congressional budget justifications.

Notes: As of February 14, 2012, the Global Fund reports having received $6.0 billion of the $6.7 billion the United States pledged to provide through FY2011. According to the Fund, the United States pledged to pay $2.7 billion in 2001-2007, $808.2 million in 2008, $1.0 billion in 2009, $1.05 billion in 2010, and $1.05 billion in 2011. See http://www.theglobalfund.org/documents/ pledges_ contributions.xls.

The $87.8 million deducted from the FY2004 total reflects language in the U.S. Leadership Against HIV/AIDS, Tuberculosis, and Malaria Act (P.L. 108-25) that prohibited U.S. contributions to the Fund from exceeding 33% of contributions from all sources (discussed below). Through the FY2005 Consolidated Appropriations (P.L. 108- 447), Congress replaced the $87.8 million and added it to the FY2005 contribution.

KEY DEVELOPMENTS WITHIN THE GLOBAL FUND

A founding principle of the Global Fund is to consistently evaluate and adapt its operations, architecture, and grants according to changing needs and circumstances. The section below highlights key developments within the Global Fund that have followed independent evaluations, feedback from various stakeholders, and discussions about misuse of Global Fund resources.

Evaluating the Global Fund

The Global Fund's Board decided at its sixth meeting in October 2003 to hire an independent team of experts to conduct a five-year evaluation of its grants.

The purpose was to ascertain the extent to which the Global Fund had reached its performance goals and adhered to its founding principles. In November 2006, the Board approved the launch of the five-year evaluation, which was overseen by Board-appointed public health experts, known as the Technical Evaluation Reference Group (TERG), and conducted between April 2007 and October 2008 by a separate team of independent consultants who assessed three key areas:

- the efficiency and effectiveness of the Global Fund's structure,
- the effectiveness and impact of the Global Fund's partnership system, and
- the impact of Global Fund grants on the three diseases.

It is important to note that independent expert teams have conducted eight different evaluations since the Fund was established, all of which have inspired reforms.

However, the five-year evaluation provided the first comprehensive assessment of the Global Fund.[16] In March 2009, the team of evaluators published its overall assessments and recommendations, which focused on

- improving the sustainability of Global Fund grants;
- sustaining spending by recipient countries on HIV/AIDS, TB, and malaria in light of increased donor spending;
- strengthening health systems;

- improving monitoring and evaluation indicators; and
- enhancing donor coordination.

Since the release of the five-year evaluation report in 2009, the Global Fund has instituted several changes based on its recommendations, and other recommendations made following additional external reviews and internal assessments. In September 2010, the Secretariat consolidated those and previously launched initiatives into a reform agenda for a more efficient and effective Global Fund.[17] At the Global Fund's 22nd Board Meeting in December 2010, the Board approved the reform agenda and established a Comprehensive Reform Working Group (CRWG) to further develop ongoing efforts and define a more comprehensive plan for Global Fund reform. At the Global Fund Board's 23rd Meeting, held in May 2011, the Board approved a series of measures recommended by the reform working group, including

- *strengthening the accountability framework*—enhancing fiduciary control and risk management, improving the tailoring of risk management approaches to local contexts, and applying stronger standards for implementers;
- *strengthening partnerships*—at the country level, introducing formal agreements on technical and management assistance and at the global level, better clarifying partnership roles;
- *enhancing value for money*—leveraging the Global Fund's market-shaping role to improve price, quality, and availability of key health products, and encourage reprogramming of funding toward more cost-effective interventions;
- *improving governance*—reviewing the Global Fund Board's governance structures and operating procedures to ensure more efficient and effective decision making; and
- *adapting the Global Fund business model*—moving from one-size-fits-all solutions to better take into account the grant performance record, implementation risks, and the extent of Global Fund support in countries relative to other health financing.

These reforms are each reaffirmed in the 2012-2016 Global Fund Strategy.

Since 2009, the Global Fund has also been developing a common platform for funding and planning programs that strengthen health systems with the Global Alliance for Vaccines and Immunization (GAVI) and World Bank.[18] The purpose of this new platform is to develop (1) common funding policies for health systems strengthening, (2) common country eligibility criteria, (3) joint review mechanisms for proposals and program oversight, (4) harmonization of technical support, and (5) a common framework for measuring performance.[19] Some of the expected benefits of the joint platform include reduced transaction costs, increased global focus on health systems strengthening, enhanced predictability of donor funding, and improved harmonization and alignment of funding and programming for health systems strengthening.[20] This platform will be implemented starting in 2014.

Addressing Corruption

On January 23, 2011, the Associated Press released an article that discussed instances of corruption discovered by the Global Fund's Inspector General's Office.[21] The article focused on allegations of corruption and fraud in 4 of the 145 countries that receive Global Fund grants: Mali, Djibouti, Mauritania, and Zambia. Shortly thereafter, both critics and supporters of the Global Fund released statements about corruption in foreign aid in general and the Global Fund's response to corruption in particular.[22] Although this is not the first time the Global Fund has uncovered misuse of funds, these recent examples may have increased scrutiny of U.S. support to the Fund, especially in an austere budget environment.

According to the Global Fund, it has a zero-tolerance policy for corruption and has taken several actions to address instances of fraud, including freezing disbursements, expenditures, and activities until measures are taken to account for funds; recovering misused funds; and changing principal recipients.[23] When the situation merits it, grants are terminated, suspended, or placed under the Global Fund's Additional Safeguard policies.

On February 4, 2011, the Global Fund announced that it had instituted several measures "to reinforce its financial safeguards and increase its capacity to prevent and detect fraud and misuse in its grants, many of which are already underway."[24] These measures included

- expanding the mandate of firms that monitor expenditure in countries in order to enhance fraud prevention and detection;
- strengthening the role of country coordinating bodies in grant oversight;
- heightening scrutiny of activities at higher risk of fraud, such as training;

- redirecting a proportion of all grants to assess and strengthen financial controls at country levels;
- increasing the number of the Fund's staff responsible for financial management; and
- doubling the budget of the Fund's independent Inspector General.[25]

In April 2011, the Senate Foreign Relations Committee released a minority report offering background information on the Global Fund and a discussion of responses taken by the Global Fund to address general corruption issues as well as this specific case.[26] The report included a number of recommendations to strengthen the oversight of Global Fund procurement procedures (see "Transparency, Monitoring, and Evaluation"). The report also noted several steps that the Fund has taken toward preventing financial mismanagement, including

- increasing the staffing and budgetary support for the Office of the Inspector General from 19 staff with a 2009 budget of $6.67 million to 30 staff positions with a proposed budget of $19.79 million for 2011; and
- establishing the Global Fund Comprehensive Reform Working Group, which is tasked with writing a report that recommends financial reforms. The Working Group consists of the Chair and Vice Chair of the Board of the Global Fund, the Executive Director of the Secretariat, three donor representatives (including the United States), and three representatives from recipient countries.

Also in April 2011, the Global Fund released a report that outlined the steps the Global Fund has taken to safeguard against misuse of funds.[27] According to the report, the Global Fund uncovered the misuse of funds in 11 countries totaling $44.2 million. About 63% of these misused funds were identified in four countries: Djibouti, Mali, Mauritania, and Zambia. An October 2011 report from the Office of the Inspector General found evidence of further misuse of funds in Nigeria. The Global Fund is reportedly seeking restitution of misused funds and has submitted evidence in support of criminal investigations in Mali, Mauritania, and Zambia.

At the Global Fund's May 2011 Board Meeting, the Fund's Office of the Inspector General (OIG) raised a number of issues the Board might consider, including the following:

- *Reconsidering the relevance of the Global Fund's model*, given the environment in which the Global Fund is often operating. The OIG proposed that the Fund reconsider whether to remain just a financing institution, reliant upon national ownership. If the Board decides to retain that model, the OIG recommends identifying other options to mitigate the risks of fraud and financial misappropriation that are currently inadequately addressed.
- *Making risk management part and parcel of the grant making process.*
- *Reevaluating the Key Performance Indicator (KPI) structure*. The OIG asserted that the KPI structure's emphasis on speed and quantity of disbursements often compromises quality and adequate consideration of risks. Further, the OIG recommended that the Board revisit the concept as an appropriate mechanism for measuring the performance of Fund Portfolio Managers and Secretariat staff. At the same time, the OIC urged the Board to consider developing tools to measure the delivery of quality products and the effective use of resources.
- *Establishing minimum acceptable capacity standards* to assess Principal Recipients and develop a system to hold Principal Recipients accountable when things go wrong.
- *Enforcing the policies and guidelines* that have not been implemented at country level.
- *Making the Country Coordinating Mechanisms more effective* in their oversight duties and ensuring that they are without conflicts of interest.[28]

Further, on June 23, 2011, the Global Fund announced that it had signed an agreement with the International Aid Transparency Initiative, a multilateral effort (including donors, countries, and civil society organizations) to publicly disclose aid data in a standardized, timely approach.[29]

In September 2011, the High-Level Independent Review Panel on Fiduciary Controls and Oversight Mechanisms of the Global Fund released a report that recommends improving financial and Board oversight, simplifying the grant application process, and putting in place better mitigation strategies to identify, assess, and manage risk.[30] In November 2011, the Global Fund Board adopted the report and its recommendations, and released the "Consolidated Transformation Plan," which outlines steps toward implementing the recommended reforms, including

- improved investment of Global Fund resources toward the highest-impact countries, interventions, and populations;
- increased efficiency and value for money in the use of Global Fund resources;
- more effective identification and management of risks;
- more efficient and flexible management of grants in a consistent, quality-assured manner;
- enhanced structure and management of the Secretariat and the Board for optimal performance;
- enhanced engagement of partners at global, regional and country levels, to support grant performance; and
- increased predictability and sustainability of funding.[31]

Reforming Financial Eligibility and Recipient Country Contribution Requirements

At the May 2011 Board meeting, the Board approved the new *Eligibility Counterpart Financing and Prioritization Policy*, which affects the way Global Fund resources are provided.[32] By implementing this new policy, the Board agreed to divide Fund resources into two accounts: the General Funding Pool and the Targeted Funding Pool. Broadly speaking, the General Funding Pool is intended for countries with large disease burdens and limited domestic resources. Roughly 90% of Global Fund resources are available through the General Funding Pool. The Targeted Funding Pool builds on the dedicated reserve for most-at-risk populations (MARPs) created in round 10, and now applies to all three diseases (but not for cross-cutting HSS proposals). Proposals in the Targeted Funding Pool will also have a predefined budget ceiling: $5 million for the first two years and $12.5 million for a five-year proposal. When submitting a grant proposal, countries must clearly indicate for which funding pool they are applying. Upper middle-income countries must be able to demonstrate an extreme disease burden to be eligible for both pools, and the programs must be focused on MARPs and/or highest impact interventions; those with a high disease burden are restricted to the Targeted Funding Pool.

In addition, the new policy provides Counterpart Financing requirements that replace the old Cost Sharing Policy, which applied only to middle-income countries. This new policy requires all recipient countries, regardless of income level, to show that the government contribution to relevant national disease programs and to overall health is increasing each year, and to report on these contributions annually. The minimum contribution each country must provide toward addressing the related disease follows the following income criteria, with lower middle-income countries split into two groups:

- low-income countries: 5%
- lower lower-middle-income countries: 20%
- upper lower-middle-income countries: 40%
- upper middle-income countries: 60%

The Global Fund Strategy 2012-2016 further articulated the Fund's intention to focus on the highest-impact countries. The Strategy states that "funding decisions are guided by considerations of potential for impact, including the global distribution of disease and key specifics of individual country situations ... for the relevant disease."[33] In November 2011, the Global Fund Board also mandated a revised application and approval process for grant renewals whereby any G-20 upper middle-income country with less than an extreme disease burden would no longer be eligible for renewal of grants.[34]

Simplifying Reporting Requirements

In 2008, at its 18th meeting, the Global Fund Board decided to revise its funding architecture to simplify its business model and harmonize its grants with those supported by recipient countries and other donors. One strategy that the Board approved was to begin funding grants through a Single Stream Agreement (SSA), whereby principal recipients will report on its activities by disease rather than by round.[35] In other words, if a PR has multiple grant agreements for a disease, the grants will be consolidated into a single agreement and the PR will report on its progress through one submission.[36] The Fund hopes that the strategy will reduce the reporting burden on grant recipients and allow countries to more easily align work plans, budgets, and targets. Adherence to the new funding architecture is voluntary for round 10 and required for future rounds. The implementation of SSA will discontinue the use of the Rolling Continuation Channel (RCC) for funding.[37]

The Board also decided at its 18th meeting to pilot a new grant proposal process known as the National Strategy Application (NSA).[38] The NSA was funded in a limited number of countries and designed to more closely align Global Fund grant proposals with national health strategies and fiscal cycles;

reduce transaction costs and paperwork for recipient countries; improve harmonization with other donors who have agreed to use the process; and encourage broad-based use and support of harmonized funding structures and processes. Countries participating in the "second wave" of NSA funding are also subject to the Transitional Funding Mechanism criteria, although these countries will be able to use the jointly assessed strategy, produced for the NSA, as the basis for their funding request for continuation of essential services.[39]

Enhancing Civil Society Participation

In 2007, the Board approved the routine use of dual-track financing, which enables grants to be managed by two primary recipients, one representing national governments and the other civil society organizations (CSOs) or the private sector. Dual-track financing is not required, though any application with one primary recipient must include a justification for not using the method.[40] The TERG and other health experts have long asserted that CSOs fill key roles in advancing global health. Such functions include advocacy, demand creation, service delivery, policy-setting, and accountability. In the long run, many observers maintain that civil society engagement facilitates sustainability of outcomes, health system strengthening, and country ownership.[41] According to the Global Fund, by the end of 2009, 84% of grants managed by CSOs either met or exceeded expectations.[42] Dual-track financing was used in 28 or the 79 proposals approved by the Technical Review Panel in the 10th funding round.[43]

Applying Debt Payments to Global Fund Grants

In 2007, the Global Fund launched an initiative called Debt2Health, through which creditors allow countries to substitute the interest payments on their debt for public health spending via the Global Fund.

By June 2011, the Global Fund had signed four agreements with two creditor countries and three beneficiary countries. The Fund anticipates that these agreements will channel $107 million to efforts to fight the three diseases.[44]

Expanding Access to Improved Anti-Malarial Medication

The Affordable Medicines Facility–malaria (AMFm) initiative, launched in April 2009, was originally proposed in a 2004 report by the U.S. Institute of Medicine and developed in consultation with the Roll Back Malaria (RBM) Partnership.[45] The initiative aims to improve access to artemisinin-based combination therapy (ACT) by negotiating lower treatment prices with drug manufacturers and supporting the proper use of the anti-malarial drug. AMFm subsidizes a significant portion of the drug, dropping the purchase price from $11 per course to less than $1. Although the AMFm initiative is managed by the Global Fund, UNITAID, Britain's Department for International Development (DFID), and other donors finance and implement the initiative separately.

Through AMFm, the Global Fund anticipates ACTs supplanting cheaper, commonly used antimalarial drugs that have high drug resistance rates. Some observers warn, however, that people could take ACTs with the onset of symptoms like fever without being diagnosed with malaria. In light of decreased efficacy of ACTs along the Thai-Cambodia border and that ACTs are the only anti-malarial drugs without widespread resistance, several health experts urge the Fund to finance rapid diagnostic tests to complement AMFm activites and prevent drug resistance to ACTs.[46]

Strengthening Supply Chain Systems

In June 2009, the Global Fund launched the Voluntary Pooled Procurement (VPP) Initiative, which encourages collective procurement of drugs and related commodities to decrease prices, expand access to quality medicines, and improve the reliability of drug supplies. The initiative focuses on four product categories: first-line antiretroviral treatment (ART), second-line ART, ACT drugs, and long-lasting insecticide treated nets (LLINs). By monitoring prices, cost savings, and market shares, the Global Fund hopes to strengthen national procurement systems and supply chain management. Between June 2009 and December 2010, the Global Fund procured goods in over 40 countries worth more than $500 million through this mechanism.[47] The Global Fund reports that additional consultations are underway in 10 more countries that have expressed interest in receiving capacity-building and supply chain management assistance.[48]

ISSUES FOR CONGRESS

Since making a founding pledge to the Fund in 2001, the United States has strongly supported the Fund: U.S. contributions have remained higher than any other country, U.S. officials have served on various Global Fund boards, and Congress has steadily raised appropriations to the Fund. At the same time, Congress has passed laws that limit U.S. spending on the Fund, such as a stipulation that prohibits U.S. contributions from exceeding one-third of all contributions.

Despite strong support by past Congresses for global health programs, including the Global Fund, some Members of Congress have begun to question U.S. spending on non-security foreign aid and argue for reducing or eliminating development and health aid. Although some Members of Congress argue that cuts to these programs could yield important savings, others contend that the cuts would have little impact on the federal deficit, while significantly imperiling the lives of vulnerable populations reliant on U.S. assistance. The section below discusses issues the 112th Congress might consider as it debates spending levels for the Global Fund.

FY2013 Budget Debate

The FY2013 budget request included $1.65 billion for the Global Fund, a significant increase from previous years in contrast to some proposed cuts in bilateral global health programs. Key questions are whether the 112th Congress will approve the proposed increase while congressional debate continues to focus on limiting government spending overall, or whether it will agree with the Administration's proportional focus on the Global Fund.

Although appropriations for the Global Fund have mostly climbed, spending for the Fund has become a declining share of total U.S. spending on international HIV/AIDS, TB, and malaria programs, particularly from FY2007 through FY2011 (*Table 3).* In FY2012, a slightly larger share of global HIV/AIDS, TB, and malaria resources went toward the Global Fund. Should Congress meet the President's request, the Fund will become an even greater share of U.S. global HIV/AIDS, TB, and malaria spending in FY2013.

Table 3. U.S. Global HIV/AIDS, TB, and Malaria Funding, FY2001-FY2013 (current U.S. $ millions)

	FY2001-FY2004 Actual	*FY2005 Actual*	*FY2006 Actual*	*FY2007 Actual*	*FY2008 Actual*	*FY2009 Actual*	*FY2010 Actual*	*FY2011 Actual*	*FY2012 Estimate*	*FY2013 Request*
U.S. Spending Global Fund	1,081.7	347.2	544.5	724.0	840.3	1,000.0	1,050.0	1,045.8	1,300.0	1,650.0
U.S. Spending										
HIV/AIDS,TB,	4,995.2	2,519.6	2,932.1	4,156.8	5,5670.6	6,193.6	6,531.4	6,464.4	6,124.7	5,535.5
Malaria										
TOTAL	6,076.9	2,866.8	3,476.6	4,880.8	6,510.9	7,193.6	7,581.4	7,510.20	7,424.7	7,185.5
Global Fund										
Share of TOTAL	*17.8%*	*12.1%*	*15.7%*	*14.8%*	*12.9%*	*13.9%*	*13.9%*	*13.9%*	*17.5%*	*23.0%*
US										

Sources: CRS analysis of appropriations legislation and congressional budget justifications.

Debate about supporting the Global Fund has often focused on HIV/AIDS. Nonetheless, some global health experts urge Congress to consider the impact of the Global Fund on the other two diseases. The Global Fund estimates that by the end of 2010, it had committed some $12 billion to HIV/AIDS programs, less than half of U.S. spending levels on related bilateral projects during the same time period. The Fund outspent the United States during this time, however, on global TB and malaria projects. The Global Fund committed over three times as much funding to TB and malaria activities than the United States.

The Global Fund estimates that the $3.6 billion that it committed to TB programs accounted for 65% of all donor spending in 2009, far exceeding the $1.1 billion in U.S. bilateral spending.[49] Advocates assert that U.S. support for the Global Fund enables the United States to invest in TB programs, an area in which the United States has a relatively limited presence. Proponents of greater spending on TB point to the dire impact of HIV/TB co-infection, particularly in sub-Saharan Africa, which has complicated efforts to control the spread of tuberculosis and accelerated the rate at which people die from either disease.

Supporters for a diversified U.S. global health portfolio also point to the role that the Global Fund plays in eliminating malaria. According to the Fund, it has committed roughly $6.1 billion to malaria programs since its inauguration, accounting for some 65% of total donor spending through the end of 2009.[50] Since the launch of the President's Malaria Initiative, U.S. investments in global malaria programs has increased substantially, though U.S. spending on malaria from FY2001 through FY2010 amounted to about one-third as much as Global Fund commitments.

Congress may also consider potential advantages of the Global Fund over U.S. bilateral health programs. Some experts argue that the Fund's grant process allows for greater country ownership of programs, more flexibility in tailoring programs to specific country priorities, and supports interventions that are better integrated with existing national and civil society activities. These experts argue that these attributes may make these programs more sustainable in the future and less dependent on U.S. assistance. Some also argue that the fund allows donors to pool and leverage their resources, reduces overlaps in programming, and has fewer overhead costs. Alternatively, others argue that the Global Fund model is more unpredictable than bilateral programs, does not allow for adequate oversight of funds, and is more difficult to track and measure.

U.S. Leadership in Combating HIV/AIDS, TB, and Malaria

The United States spends more on combating HIV/AIDS than any other country and is a key donor for international malaria and TB programs. Experts continue to debate whether the United States should maintain that leadership, including, in particular, the level to which the United States should be a leader in supporting the Global Fund.

U.S. Spending Ceilings

Many urge Congress to increase appropriations to the Fund, in large part because donors have begun to follow the lead of the United States in setting their annual contributions. However, U.S. contributions to the Fund cannot exceed 33% of all contributions, a condition first set through the U.S. Leadership Against HIV/AIDS, Tuberculosis, and Malaria Act (P.L. 108-25). The law that extended the authorization of U.S. support to the Fund, the Tom Lantos and Henry J. Hyde United States Global Leadership Against HIV/AIDS, Tuberculosis, and Malaria Reauthorization Act of 2008 (P.L. 110-293), maintained this requirement. Many observers speculate that Congress instituted the contribution limit to encourage greater global support for the Fund. For this reason, some argue that U.S. ceiling should remain. As of yet, it does not look like the FY2013 request, if approved, would exceed this spending ceiling.

U.S. Share of Donor Contributions

Advocates of the Fund argue that U.S. support for the Fund has become even more important since the global financial crisis. The Global Fund announced in November 2009 that it would reduce the budgets of grants approved in round 9 by 10% for the first two years, and by 25% for the subsequent years.[51] In 2010, the Global Fund published a report that outlined various resource scenarios and the Fund's resulting ability to approve new grants. The Fund estimated that it would need between $13 billion and $20 billion from 2011 to 2013 to maintain programs, and upwards of $20 billion to scale-up efforts.[52]

Donors met for two days starting on October 4, 2010, at the United Nations headquarters in New York City to pledge their support for the next three years of the Global Fund.[53] The Global Fund announced on October 5, 2010, that the international community had pledged to provide some $11.7 billion to the Global Fund over the next three years, roughly $1 billion less than the Global Fund's most conservative funding request. The U.S. pledge accounted for roughly 34% ($4 billion) of that amount. Subsequent pledges totaling $11.8 million by Luxembourg ($10.8 million) and Rwanda ($1 million) were made following the pledging conference.[54]

In November 2011, the Global Fund announced that, due to inadequate resources from donors, it would cancel its 11th round of funding and would not be supporting any new grants until 2014.[55] Some experts argue that the lack of new funding from the Global Fund during this time period could have dire consequences. As the largest donor in the world for TB and malaria efforts, and a key player in the fight against HIV/AIDS, many believe that a reduction in Global Fund grants could significantly undercut the potential for progress against these three diseases.[56]

Despite concerns about the Global Fund's ability to finance qualified grants from developing countries, some observers would like the Global Fund to address its own capacity before urging Congress to increase support for the organization.[57]

Coordinating the Global Fund with U.S. Global Health Programs

Since the Global Fund was launched, the United States has sought to better coordinate Global Fund and related bilateral programs. Through the Global Health Initiative (GHI), the Obama Administration has affirmed its intention to increase cooperation with the Fund, indicating that one of the seven basic principles of GHI is to "strengthen and leverage key multilateral organizations, global health partnerships and private sector engagement" with the purpose of implementing a coordinated strategy across other major donors and national governments.[58] In its Five-Year Strategy report, the Office of the Global AIDS Coordinator (OGAC) emphasized its partnership with the Global Fund and outlined several steps to ensure the Fund's long-term sustainability, including transferring some PEPFAR programs to the Global Fund and coordinating and aligning activities related to the funding, monitoring, and evaluation of PEPFAR, Global Fund, and UNAIDS programs.[59]

Many observers question the strength of the U.S. commitment to donor coordination. For example, though U.S. representatives have advocated better alignment of project implementation, a common framework for such a notion has yet to be formalized. The Global Fund has begun to develop a joint funding platform for health systems strengthening with other groups, however, like GAVI, the World Bank, and WHO. Though the United States is not party to the platform, OGAC has expressed limited support for the undertaking.[60] Despite OGAC's support for increased coordination among donors of health system strengthening efforts, it also contended that each donor has a unique mandate and role to play in strengthening health systems. WHO and other health experts urge key donors, including the United States, to align reporting and auditing requirements, the frequency and type of data collected and reported, and fiscal cycles in an effort to reduce the transaction costs and staffing requirements of recipient countries.[61]

Transparency, Monitoring, and Evaluation

Some critics of the Fund contend that the Fund's oversight mechanisms are not strong enough to protect against wasteful spending, particularly in countries that have a well-documented history of corruption and poor financial management. Fund supporters counter that the release of evaluations and findings on the Global Fund's website reflect the Fund's commitment to reporting and monitoring its projects. Specifically, the Fund has uploaded onto its website an abundance of information on grant proposals and budgets, grant spending trends, and results of board meetings, which include decisions regarding the suspension of grants. Fund advocates also argue that the Fund's decisions to suspend temporarily and, in some cases, discontinue poor performing grants demonstrate the effectiveness of the Fund's oversight and funding mechanisms.

Some in Congress have long advocated for stronger oversight of Global Fund spending. Supporters of this idea have welcomed language included in FY2006 and FY2008 foreign operations appropriations measures, which required the Secretary of State to withhold up to 20% of the U.S. contribution to the Global Fund until she determined the Fund had adhered to U.S. reporting and monitoring standards. In FY2009, the withholding was reduced to 10%. Beginning in the FY2010 foreign operations appropriations, the Lantos-Hyde Act (P.L. 110-293), which authorized the extension of PEPFAR programs and funding for U.S. bilateral TB and malaria programs, required the Secretary of State to withhold 20% of the U.S. contribution to the Global Fund until she certified that the Fund had met requirements pertaining to the Local Fund Agent (LFA) performance, a policy of transparency, an independent Office of the Inspector General, and several other policy and procedural provisions.

Most recently, the FY2012 foreign operations appropriations included language requiring the Secretary of State to withhold up to 10% of Global Fund support until she determined that the Fund was implementing a policy of transparency, supporting an independent Office of the Inspector General, and maintaining an effective whistleblower policy to protect whistleblowers from retaliation.[62] To date, the U.S. government has not withheld funds on the basis of any of the above provisions. The Global AIDS Coordinator has signed this certification, on behalf of the Secretary of State under delegated authority, in past years. The State Department will report to Congress on the FY2012 provision after the fiscal year reporting period has ended in September 2012.

Some Global Fund supporters contend, however, that such action is unnecessary in light of the consistent release of information by the Global Fund on grant performance and funding. Global Fund advocates point to actions by the Global Fund to release information on discoveries of fraud despite the negative press reports that surfaced in early 2011, as well as subsequent steps taken to suspend or transfer management of relevant grants.[63] Some experts applaud the Global Fund's efforts in this area and urge the United States to release similar information on the performance and funding of its bilateral health programs.[64]

In light of the vigorous debate regarding responses by the Global Fund to corruption, a number of recommendations made by the Senate Foreign Relations Committee's minority staff to strengthen the oversight of Global Fund grants in particular and U.S. global health spending in general may receive attention in the 112th Congress.[65] These included calls to:

1. Make U.S. contributions to the Global Fund contingent upon the Global Fund Boards' adoption of reforms laid out by the U.S. Department of State. The Department of State would be required to certify to Congress that the reforms were in place before funds could be released.
2. Withhold all funding to UNDP until it certifies that its internal rules and procedures have been sufficiently modified to allow the Inspector General of the Global Fund, the Inspector General of the World Bank, and any investigative arm of any multilateral organization to which the United States contributes funds full access to their audits, investigations, records, and personnel.
3. Withhold U.S. contributions from the Global Fund to the UNDP until the United States receives confirmation of such certification.

4. Instruct the Government Accountability Office to conduct a study regarding the coordination of the Office of Inspectors General (or equivalent offices) of all U.S. government entities and multilateral organizations receiving U.S. taxpayer funds that oversee the integrity of global health programs.
5. Have the U.S. Representative to the Global Fund reiterate in the strongest terms to the Board of the Global Fund that the United States has no tolerance for fraud and abuse and that the Office of the Inspector General needs to acquire adequate resources and personnel to audit and investigate programs on the ground.
6. Have the Global Fund take any steps necessary to ensure that Local Fund Agents and CCMs are capable of managing grants and are properly trained on how to spot and mitigate suspected fraudulent activities.
7. Have the U.S. government conduct a top-to-bottom analysis of U.S. investment and contributions to international organizations and funds, similar to that conducted by Britain. On March 1, 2011, the United Kingdom Department for International Development issued a Multilateral Review, which evaluated the 43 international funds and organizations that the United Kingdom contributes with respect to value for the money and each fund's and organization's effectiveness in combating poverty, taking in account transparency and accountability.[66]
8. Have the U.S. government work more closely with host governments on establishing or increasing the country's commitment to making its own investments in health programs. When possible, the countries must demonstrate some commitment in moving toward sustainability and cease complete reliance on the donor community for the indefinite future.

Since the release of this report, the Global Fund has announced several plans to increase transparency, monitoring, and evaluation of its programs, particularly through the Consolidated Transformation Plan.

CONCLUSION

To date, the Global Fund has approved funding for over 1,000 projects in 150 countries. Through its treatment, prevention, and care efforts, the Fund estimates that it has saved approximately 7.7 million lives. Despite these achievements, observers raise several issues that could influence U.S. support for the Fund:

- *The appropriate balance between U.S. support for the Global Fund and bilateral HIV/AIDS, TB, and malaria programs*—Since the Global Fund was created, some have weighed U.S. contributions to the Global Fund against U.S. spending on bilateral HIV/AIDS, TB, and malaria efforts. The Office of the Global AIDS Coordinator rejects this notion and presents the Global Fund as a complement to U.S. bilateral programs. Nonetheless, the 112th Congress will likely debate the distribution of U.S. support between the Global Fund and related bilateral programs, especially PEPFAR.[67] The President's FY2013 budget request may contribute to this debate, as it proposes decreased funding for bilateral HIV/AIDS, TB, and malaria programs while proposing increased funding for the Global Fund. Some experts argue that this reflects the relative efficient and flexible nature of multilateral programs. Others argue that increasing funding for the Fund while decreasing funding for bilateral programs undercuts the success of more predictable and sustainable U.S. programs.
- *How to coordinate Global Fund and bilateral HIV/AIDS, TB, and malaria programs*—When President Obama announced GHI, he expressed his intent to reshape U.S. global health policy so that global health efforts were better integrated and coordinated. Despite references throughout the GHI Implementation Plan to stronger collaboration with the Global Fund, the extent to which such an effort will occur is not yet clear. While several official U.S. documents support calls from the Global Fund to enhance donor coordination, the United States has expressed limited support for a joint funding platform for health systems strengthening.[68] U.S. officials maintain each donor has a unique mandate and role to play.[69]
- *Growing emphasis on improving health systems*—Despite calls by the Global Fund for more financial support, the team of experts who conducted a five-year evaluation of the Fund warned that recipient

countries might not be able to continue receiving assistance at current scale without significant investments in health systems.[70] The Global Fund and other donors have increased spending on improving global health systems, nonetheless challenges in this area persist. One of the goals of the Global Health Initiative is to improve health systems through several strategies, such as addressing health system bottlenecks, strengthening data collection systems, improving human resources for health, and donor coordination.[71] Several global health experts recommend that the Global Fund and other donors support national health plans and address the major gaps in basic health service availability and readiness as part of HIV/AIDS, TB, and malaria efforts.

- *Whether Global Fund resources should be used in middle-income countries*—Several observers question the use of Global Fund resources in middle-income countries. In 2010, 11 countries were considered both donors and recipients: China, India, Malaysia, Namibia, Nigeria, Romania, Rwanda, Russia, South Africa, Thailand, and Tunisia.[72] China has received the most attention from all of these countries, due to both the substantial amount of grants it has received from the Fund and the rapid growth of its economy. The Global Fund awards grants to lower middle-income countries, but expects them to contribute up to program costs. For example, as a middle-income country with a per capita income of $3,650 China is eligible for Global Fund grants and pays roughly 80% of total program costs.[73] The Senate Foreign Relations Committee's minority report recommends that as China becomes an upper middle-income country, it should no longer receive Global Fund resources. In May 2011, the Global Fund approved a new Eligibility, Counterpart Financing and Prioritization Policy that limits how much funding middle-income countries could receive through the Fund and requires all countries to contribute to national disease and health strategies and demonstrate increased funding for these activities annually. At the November 2011 board meeting, the Global Fund also implemented a policy whereby G-20 upper middle-income countries will no longer be eligible for grant renewals unless they have an extreme disease burden, as defined by the Fund.
- *The Fund's responses to allegations of corruption*—The Global Fund's announcement that funds from some its grants were misspent has opened a rigorous debate in the foreign aid community. Some

observers applauded the Global Fund for its transparency and encouraged others to release similar information, arguing that the Global Fund is not alone in facing these problems. Advocates also note efforts by the Fund to reform its fiduciary practices and reduce corruption. On the other hand, some have called for governments to withhold support for the Global Fund until adequate safeguards are established. The Global Fund's release of information on misused funds by its grant recipients raises several questions. If the Global Fund is penalized for being honest in its shortcomings, will others hesitate to do so? When allegations of corruption and malfeasance are discovered, what is the appropriate response? What impact might reduced funding have on those relying on aid programs for life-saving treatments?

APPENDIX. ACRONYMS AND INITIALISMS

3D Fund	Three Diseases Fund
AMFm	Affordable Medicine Facility–malaria
ACT	Artemisinin-based Combination drug Treatment
ART	Antiretroviral Therapy
CBJ	Congressional Budget Justification
CCM	Country Coordinating Mechanism
CDC	U.S. Centers for Disease Control and Prevention
CGD	Center for Global Development
CSO	Civil Society Organization
DOD	U.S. Department of Defense
DOL	U.S. Department of Labor
DOTS	Directly Observed Treatment Short-Course
EU	European Union
GAO	U.S. Government Accountability Office
GAVI	Global Alliance for Vaccines and Immunization
GHI	Global Health Initiative
HHS	U.S. Department of Health and Human Services
HSS	Health System Strengthening
IRS	Indoor Residual Spraying
ITN	Insecticide-Treated Net
LFA	Local Funding Agent
LLIN	Long Lasting Insecticide-treated Nets

MDG	Millennium Development Goals
MDR-TB	Multi-Drug Resistant Tuberculosis
NGO	Non-Governmental Organization
NSA	National Strategy Application
NTD	Neglected Tropical Diseases
OGAC	Office of the Global AIDS Coordinator
PEPFAR	President's Emergency Plan for AIDS Relief
PMTCT	Prevention of Mother To Child HIV Transmission
PR	Principal Recipient
RBM	Roll Back Malaria
RCC	Rolling Continuation Channel
SR	Sub-recipient
SSA	Single Stream Agreement
TB	Tuberculosis
TERG	Technical Evaluation Reference Group
UN	United Nations
UNAIDS	Joint United Nations Program on HIV/AIDS
UNDP	United Nations Development Program
USAID	U.S. Agency for International Development
VCT	Voluntary Counseling and Testing
VPP	Voluntary Pooled Procurement
WHO	World Health Organization

End Notes

[1] See Global Fund, The Framework Document of the Global Fund to Fight AIDS, Tuberculosis, and Malaria, 2001, http://www.theglobalfund.org/documents/TGF_Framework.pdf.

[2] For background information on the Global Fund and its structure, see CRS Report RL31712, The Global Fund to Fight AIDS, Tuberculosis, and Malaria: Background, by Tiaji Salaam-Blyther.

[3] Global Fund, Report of the Technical Review Panel and the Secretariat on Round 10 Proposals, December 13-15, 2010, http://www.theglobalfund.org/documents/board/ 22/BM22_13 TRPRound10_Report_en.pdf.

[4] Global Fund website, Grant Portfolio, accessed on February 13, 2012, http://portfolio.theglobalfund.org/.

[5] Global Fund, Making a Difference: Global Fund Results Report, May 2011, p. 4, http://www.theglobalfund.org/ documents/publications/progress_reports/Publication_2011Results_Report_en.pdf.

[6] Global Fund, "Global Fund Welcomes U.S. Secretary of State Hillary Clinton's Support for Global Fund," press release, November 9, 2011, http://www.theglobalfund.org/fr/media center/pressreleases/2011-11-09; and Global Fund, "Global Fund Supported Programs See

Strong Results Amid Funding Challenges," press release, November 30, 2011, http://www.theglobalfund.org/en/mediacenter/pressreleases/2011-11-30.

[7] Global Fund, Transitional Funding Mechanism (TFM) Information Note, December 12, 2011.

[8] Global Fund, The Global Fund Strategy 2012-2016: Investing for Impact, November 2011.

[9] Global Fund, Consolidated Transformation Plan, Twenty-Fifth Board Meeting, November 21-22, 2011.

[10] Turning the Page from Emergency to Sustainability, The Final Report of the High-Level Independent Review Panel on Fiduciary Controls and Oversight Mechanisms of the Global Fund to Fight AIDS, Tuberculosis and Malaria, September 19, 2011.

[11] The Office of the Inspector General was established by the Board of the Global Fund to Fight AIDS, Tuberculosis, and Malaria in July 2005. The Office of the Inspector General operates as an independent unit of the Global Fund, reporting directly to the Board. The Office of the Inspector General provides the Global Fund with independent and objective assurance over the design and effectiveness of controls in place to manage the key risks impacting the Global Fund's programs and operations.

[12] Unless otherwise indicated, information in this section was taken from Global Fund, Performance-Based Funding at the Global Fund, November 2009, http://www.theglobalfund.org/documents/performance/Performancebased_Funding_brochure.pdf, and the Global Fund website, Performance-Based Funding at the Global Fund, http://www.theglobalfund.org/ en/performancebasedfunding/grantlifecycle/, February 2012.

[13] If a grant is terminated, the Global Fund ensures that lifesaving treatments are continuously dispersed for up to 21 months under the Global Fund's Continuation of Services policy. This policy was invoked to give countries sufficient time to find replacement funding and to avoid treatment interruptions, which can lead to death or drug resistance.

[14] See Department of State, "Statement by Ambassador Eric Goosby, U.S. Global AIDS Coordinator, U.S. Department of State, on the Appointment of the Global Fund Independent Review Panel Co-Chairs," press release, March 16, 2011, http://www.pepfar.gov/ press/releases/2011/158413.htm.

[15] U.S. Congress, House Committee on Appropriations, Subcommittee on State, Foreign Operations, and Related Programs, FY2012, 112th Cong., 1st sess., March 31, 2011.

[16] Evaluations overseen by the TERG include (1) Assessment of the Country Coordinating Mechanisms (CCMs); (2) Assessment of the Proposal Development and Review Process; (3) 360 Degree Stakeholder Assessment; (4) Global Fund Portfolio Review; (5) Evaluation of the Local Fund Agent System; (6) Five Year Evaluation Study Area 1: Global Fund Organizational Efficiency & Effectiveness; (7) Five Year Evaluation Study Area 2: Global Fund Partner Environment; and (8) Five Year Evaluation Study Area 3: Health Impact of Scaling Up Against HIV, TB & Malaria; Links to all evaluation materials for the studies overseen by the TERG can be found at http://www.theglobalfund.org/en/terg/

[17] For further details on the reforms, see Global Fund, An Agenda for a More Efficient and Effective Global Fund, September 2010, http://www.theglobalfund.org/documents/replenishment/2010/.

[18] Global Fund, Making a Difference: Global Fund Results Report, May 2011, p. 77.

[19] World Bank, GAVI, Global Fund and WHO, "Work Plan for 2010 Health Systems Funding Platform," March 2, 2010, http://siteresources.worldbank.org/INTHSD/Resources/topics/415176-1251914777461/ HealthSystemsFundignPlatformWorkPlanMarch22010.pdf.

[20] Global Fund, Global Fund 2010 Innovation and Impact, Progress Report 2010, p. 88.

[21] John Heilprin, "Fraud Plagues Global Health Fund Backed by Bono, Others," Associated Press, January 23, 2011, http://www.msnbc.msn.com/id/41221202/ns/health-health_care/.

[22] Kaiser Family Foundation, AP Reports On Global Fund Grant Money Lost To Corruption, Global Fund Responds, January 25, 2011, http://globalhealth.kff.org/Daily-Reports /2011/January/25/GH-012511-Global-Fund.aspx; Roger Bate, Transparency and the Global Fund's Healthy Crisis, American Enterprise Institute for Public Policy Research, February 3, 2011, http://www.aei.org/speech/100188; and Michael Gerson, "Putting Fraud Into Context," Washington Post, February 4, 2011, http://www.washingtonpost.com/wp-dyn/content/article/2011/02/03/AR2011020305176.html.

[23] For more information, see Global Fund, Results With Integrity: The Global Fund's Response to Fraud, April 2011, http://www.theglobalfund.org/documents/core/ white papers /Core_ ResultsWithIntegrityResponseToFraud_WhitePaper_en.pdf.

[24] Global Fund, "Statement by the Board Chair and Vice-Chair," press release, February 8, 2011, http://www.theglobalfund.org/en/announcements/?an=an_110209.

[25] Critics of Global Fund's fiduciary practices have also raised questions about whether the United Nations Development Program (UNDP) had established adequate protections against corruption. UNDP oversees roughly 12% of Global Fund grants, primarily in countries emerging from natural disasters, conflicts, or political crises. Detractors were particularly concerned about allegations that the data UNDP submitted was not comprehensive enough and prevented Global Fund's auditors from conducting thorough financial assessments. UNDP announced on February 4, 2011, that it had enhanced its fiduciary mechanisms and that it had taken several steps to strengthen the oversight of its funds, including recruiting dedicated and specialized fulltime investigators to respond to credible allegations of fraud or corruption in UNDP-managed Global Fund grants; developing formal "capacity development" initiatives in all countries where UNDP manages Global Fund grants; allowing the Global Fund to access UNDP audit reports of Global Fund projects, a privilege currently restricted to UN Member States; and signing a Memorandum of Understanding between UNDP's Office of Audit and Investigation and the Global Fund's Office of the Inspector-General to strengthen co-operation and information-sharing on investigations into fraud and corruption.

[26] U.S. Congress, Senate Committee on Foreign Relations, Fraud and Abuse of Global Fund Investments at Risk Without Greater Transparency, committee print, A Minority Staff Report, 112th Cong., 1st sess., April 5, 2011, S. Prt. 112-17.

[27] For more information, see Global Fund, Results With Integrity: The Global Fund's Response to Fraud, April 2011.

[28] Global Fund, The Office of the Inspector General Progress Report for November 2010-March 2011, 23rd Board Meeting, May 11-12, 2011, pp. 8-9, http://www.theglobalfund.org/ documents/board/23/.

[29] Global Fund, Global Fund Signs International Aid Transparency Initiative, press release, June 23, 2011, http://www.theglobalfund.org/en/pressreleases/?pr=an_110623. For more information on IATI, see http://www.aidtransparency.net/.

[30] The High-Level Independent Review Panel on Fiduciary Controls and Oversight Mechanisms of the Global Fund to Fight AIDS, Tuberculosis, and Malaria, Turning the Page from Emergency to Sustainability, September 19, 2011, http://www.theglobalfund. org/en/highlevelpanel/report/.

[31] Global Fund, Consolidated Transformation Plan, November 21, 2011, http://www.the globalfund.org/en/board/ meetings/twentyfifth/.

[32] Information about the new financing policies were compiled by CRS from Global Fund, Report of the 22nd Board Meeting, presented at the 23rd Board Meeting, May 11-12, 2011, p. 35, http://www.theglobalfund.org/documents/board/ 23/BM23_02TwentySecond Board

Meeting_Report_en.pdf, and Global Fund, Policy on Eligibility Criteria, Counterpart Financing Requirements, and Prioritization of Proposals for Funding from the Global Fund, presented at the 23rd Board Meeting, May 11-12, 2011, http://www.theglobalfund.org/documents/board/23/BM23_14PICPSCJEligibilityAttachment1_Policy_en.pdf.

33 Global Fund, The Global Fund Strategy 2012-2016: Investing for Impact, November 2011, http://www.theglobalfund.org/en/about/strategy/.

34 Global Fund, Twenty-Fifth Board Meeting Decision Points, November 21-22, 2011, http://www.theglobalfund.org/ en/board/meetings/twentyfifth/.

35 Global Fund, Twentieth Board Meeting Decision Points, November 9-11, 2009, http://www1.theglobalfund.org/ documents/board/20/GF-BM20-DecisionPoints_en.pdf.

36 Global Fund, New Grant Architecture Concept Note, March 2010, http://www.the globalfund.org/documents/ grantarchitecture/Architecture_High_Level_Concept_Note_en.pdf.

37 In November 2006, the Board established the Rolling Continuation Channel (RCC). This funding channel, which began in March 2007, permits Country Coordinating Mechanisms (CCMs) to request additional funding for grants that are performing well but set to expire. The application process for the RCC is not as rigorous as the Round process. RCC-approved grants can receive support for up to an additional six years, with the funds being awarded in three-year intervals. The channel is intended only for those grants that have demonstrated a significant contribution "to a national effort that has had, or has the potential to have in the near future, a measurable impact on the burden of the relevant disease." Global Fund, Report on the Final Decisions of the Fourteenth Board Meeting, October 31-November 3, 2006, at http://www.theglobalfund.org/en/files/boardmeeting14/GF-BM-14_Final_Decisions.pdf, visited January 16, 2008.

38 For more information on the NSA, see Global Fund, Report of the Technical Review Panel and the Secretariat on funding recommendations for National Strategy Applications of the First Learning Wave, Twentieth Board Meeting, November 9, 2009, http://www.the globalfund.org/documents/board/20/GF-BM20-11_TRP_ReportToBoard.pdf.

39 Global Fund, Participating in the Second Wave of NSAs, http://www. the global fund.org/en/nsa/participating/.

40 Report of the Policy and Strategy Committee, Global Fund Fifteenth Board Meeting, April 2007, http://www.theglobalfund.org/documents/board/15/GF-BM15-06_ReportPSC.pdf.

41 Rifat Atun et al., "Venice Statement on global health initiatives and health systems," The Lancet, vol. 374, no. 9692 (September 5, 2009), p. 784.

42 Global Fund, Global Fund 2010 Innovation and Impact, Progress Report 2010, p. 47. In assessing its grants, the Global Fund rates the performance of each based on their achievement of pre-established goals and targets. "A1" connotes exceeding expectations, "A2" meets expectations, "B1" adequate, "B2" inadequate but potential demonstrated, "C" unacceptable. Eighty-four percent of CSO-managed grants are rated A1, A2, or B1. For more on performance ratings, see http://www.theglobalfund.org/cn/ performancebase dfunding/methodology/?lang=cn.

43 Global Fund, Making a Difference: Global Fund Results Report, May 2011, p. 58.

44 Global Fund website, "Debt2Health," http://www.theglobalfund.org/en/innova tivefinancing/ debt2health/.

45 The RBM Partnership was launched in 1998 by WHO, the United Nations Children's Fund (UNICEF), the United Nations Development Program (UNDP), and the World Bank to provide a coordinated global response to the disease. Roughly 500 partners are engaged in the initiative. For more on the initiative, see http://www.rollbackmalaria.org/.

46 See WHO, "WHO releases new malaria guidelines for treatment and procurement of medicines," press release, March 9, 2010, http://www.who.int/mediacentre/news/releases/ 2010/malaria_20100308/en/; Rachel Nugent, Emma Back, and Alexandra Beith, The Race Against Drug Resistance, CGD, 2010, http://www.cgdev.org/files/ 1424207_file_CGD_ DRWG_FINAL.pdf; and Mohga Kamal-Yanni, "Affordable medicines facility for malaria: reasonable or rash?" The Lancet, vol. 375, no. 9709 (January 9, 2010), p. 121.

47 Global Fund website, "Procurement Support Services," http://www.theglobalfund.org/ en/procurement/vpp/.

48 Ibid.

49 Global Fund, Making a Difference: Global Fund Results Report, May 2011, p. 40.

50 Ibid.

51 Global Fund, Twentieth Board Meeting, Board Decisions, November 9-11, 2009, http://www.theglobalfund.org/ documents/board/20/GF-BM20-DecisionPoints_en.pdf.

52 Global fund, Resource Scenarios 2011-2013: Funding the Global Fight against HIV/AIDS, Tuberculosis and Malaria, The Global Fund Third Replenishment (2011-2013), March 2010.

53 For more details on the pledging conference, see http://www.theglobalfund.org/en/ replenishment/hague/documents/.

54 Global Fund, "Luxembourg Commits EUR 7.5 Million to the Global Fund," press release, October 27, 2010, http://www.theglobalfund.org/en/pressreleases/?pr=pr_101027; and Global Fund, "Rwanda Donates $1 million to the Global Fund," press release, November 10, 2010, http://www.theglobalfund.org/en/pressreleases/?pr=pr_101110. CRS used a currency conversion rate of 7.5€ per U.S. dollar for the Luxembourg pledge.

55 Global Fund, "The Global Fund Adopts New Strategy to Save 10 Million Lives by 2016," press release, November 23, 2011, http://www.theglobalfund.org/en/media center/ press releases/2011-11-23_The_Global_Fund_adopts_new_strategy_to_save_ 10_million_lives_by_2016/.

56 For example, see Paul Farmer, "Why the Global Fund Matters," New York Times, February 1, 2012, and International HIV/AIDS Alliance, Don't Stop Now: How Underfunding the Global Fund to Fight AIDS, Tuberculosis, and Malaria Impacts on the HIV/AIDS Response, 2012, http://www.aidsalliance.org/includes/Publication/ Alliance%20global% 20fund%20report_V6.pdf.

57 Macro International, Inc., The Five-Year Evaluation of the Global Fund to Fight AIDS, Tuberculosis, and Malaria: Synthesis of Study Areas 1, 2 and 3, March 2009, p. 21.

58 USAID, Implementation of the Global Health Initiative, Consultation Document, pp. 6-7, http://www.usaid.gov/ our_work/global_health/home/Publications/docs/ghi_consultation_document.pdf.

59 OGAC, The U.S. President's Emergency Plan for AIDS Relief, Five Year Strategy, Annex: PEPFAR and the Global Context of HIV, December 2009, pp. 13 and 16, http://www. pepfar.gov/documents/organization/133436.pdf.

60 OGAC, U.S. Government Positions on Decision Points for the Twentieth Board Meeting of the Global Fund, http://www.pepfar.gov/documents/organization/134924.pdf.

61 WHO Maximizing Positive Synergies Collaborative Group, "An assessment of interactions between global health initiatives and country health systems," The Lancet, vol. 373, no. 9681 (June 20, 2009).

62 Consolidated Appropriations Act, 2010, P.L. 112-74.

63 For example, see Global Fund, "The Global Fund Suspends AIDS Grant in Mali," press release, March 2, 2011, http://www.theglobalfund.org/en/pressreleases/?pr=pr_110302, and

Global Fund, "Global Fund to Transfer Management of HIV Grant in Mali," press release, October 19, 2011, http://www.theglobalfund.org/en/mediacenter/ pressreleases/2011-10-19_Global_Fund_to_transfer_management_of_HIV_grant_in_Mali/.

[64] Since the launch of PEPFAR, the United States has become the world's largest donor to global HIV/AIDS programs. Little is known, however, about the performance of PEPFAR programs and whether the U.S. Inspector General's Office has uncovered any misuse of funds. For more discussion on this, see, Chunling Lu et al., "Absorptive capacity and disbursements by the Global Fund to Fight AIDS, Tuberculosis and Malaria: analysis of grant implementation," The Lancet, vol. 368, no. 9534 (August 5, 2006), pp. 487-488; Nandini Oommann, What Can We Learn from the Global Fund's "Massive Fraud"? Center for Global Development, January 25, 2011, http://blogs.cgdev.org/ globalhealth/ 2011/01/what-can-we-learn-from-the-global-fund%E2%80%99s-%E2%80%9Cmassive-fraud%E2%80%9D.php.

[65] See U.S. Congress, Senate Committee on Foreign Relations, Fraud and Abuse of Global Fund Investments at Risk Without Greater Transparency, committee print, A Minority Staff Report, 112th Cong., 1st sess., April 5, 2011, S. Prt. 112-17.

[66] Following the review, Britain reaffirmed its commitment to the Global Fund and considered it "very good value for the U.K. taxpayer." See, U.K. Department of International Development, Statement by the Secretary of State for International Development: the Bilateral and Multilateral Aid Reviews, Oral Statement to the House of Commons, March 1, 2011, http://www.dfid.gov.uk/Media-Room/Speeches-and-articles/2011/BAR-MAR-oral-statement/.

[67] See question posed by Honorable Charlie Dent at U.S. Congress, House Committee on Appropriations, Subcommittee on State, Foreign Operations, and Related Programs, Global Health and HIV/AIDS Programs, 112th Cong., 1st sess., March 31, 2011.

[68] OGAC, U.S. Government Positions on Decision Points for the Twentieth Board Meeting of the Global Fund, http://www.pepfar.gov/documents/organization/134924.pdf.

[69] Ibid.

[70] Macro International, Inc., The Five-Year Evaluation of the Global Fund to Fight AIDS, Tuberculosis, and Malaria: Synthesis of Study Areas 1, 2 and 3, March 2009, p. 21.

[71] Department of State, Implementation of the Global Health Initiative: Consultation Document, February 1, 2010, pp. 14-16, http://www.pepfar.gov/documents/organization/136504.pdf.

[72] For more information on the Global Fund's policy for supporting middle-income countries, see Global Fund, Counterpart Financing, http://www.theglobalfund.org/en/application/ process/counterpartfinancing/?lang=en.

[73] U.S. Congress, Senate Committee on Foreign Relations, Fraud and Abuse of Global Fund Investments at Risk Without Greater Transparency, committee print, prepared by A Minority Staff Report, 112th Cong., 1st sess., April 5, 2011, S. Prt. 112-17.

In: United States' Global Health Assistance ISBN: 978-1-62948-387-0
Editors: Kurk B. Weller

Chapter 4

U.S. RESPONSE TO THE GLOBAL THREAT OF MALARIA: BASIC FACTS*

Alexandra E. Kendall

SUMMARY

In 2010, malaria infected an estimated 216 million people and killed 655,000 people, most of whom were children under the age of five in sub-Saharan Africa. Despite the current burden of disease, malaria is preventable and treatable. Congress has increasingly recognized malaria as an important foreign policy issue, and the United States has become a major player in the global response to the disease. In its second session, the 112th Congress will likely debate the appropriate funding levels and optimum strategy for addressing the continued challenge of global malaria.

Congress has enacted several key pieces of legislation related to global malaria control. These include the Assistance for International Malaria Control Act of 2000 (P.L. 106-570); the U.S. Leadership Against HIV/AIDS, Tuberculosis, and Malaria Act of 2003 (P.L. 108-25); and the Tom Lantos and Henry J. Hyde United States Global Leadership Against HIV/AIDS, Tuberculosis, and Malaria Reauthorization Act of 2008 (P.L. 110-293). These acts have authorized funds to be used in the fight against malaria and have shaped the ways in which U.S. malaria programs are

* This is an edited, reformatted and augmented version of a Congressional Research Service publication, CRS Report for Congress R41644, prepared for Members and Committees of Congress, from www.crs.gov, dated June 15, 2012.

coordinated and managed, including through the creation of the U.S. Global Malaria Coordinator at the United States Agency for International Development (USAID). In 2005, in response to growing international calls for global malaria control and to the success of the President's Emergency Plan for AIDS Relief (PEPFAR), President George W. Bush launched the President's Malaria Initiative (PMI), which aims to halve the burden of malaria morbidity and mortality in 70% of at-risk populations in sub-Saharan Africa by 2014. PMI brought significant new attention and funding to U.S. malaria programs and made the United States one of the largest donors for malaria efforts. While U.S. funding for global malaria programs has increased each fiscal year since FY2004, support for malaria interventions increased most precipitously beginning in FY2007 as PMI has expanded into new countries. President Obama has continued to support PMI through the Global Health Initiative (GHI).

There is evidence that the growing international response to malaria has had some success in controlling the epidemic. Since 2000, global malaria incidence has decreased by 17% and malaria mortality by 26%. Since 2000, 43 countries have reported a reduction in reported malaria cases of more than 50%, including eight African countries that have experienced 50% reduction in either confirmed malaria cases or malaria admissions and deaths. The decreases in each of these African countries are associated with intense malaria control activities. Despite these successes, several key issues pose challenges to an effective scale-up of the response to malaria. First, increasing reports of drug-resistant malaria in Southeast Asia and insecticide-resistant mosquitoes, largely in Africa, threaten the success of malaria control programs. Second, weak health systems, including shortages in health care personnel and inadequate supply chain networks, have limited the delivery of essential commodities for malaria control. There is also debate within the global health community over whether malaria efforts should increasingly target areas where malaria elimination is possible or whether efforts should remain concentrated on malaria control.

This report outlines basic facts related to global malaria, including characteristics of the epidemic and U.S. legislation, programs, funding, and partnerships related to the global response to malaria.

INTRODUCTION

The United States has supported anti-malaria programs since the 1950s. Global malaria received greater attention in 2005 when President Bush launched the President's Malaria Initiative (PMI), a five-year plan to expand U.S. malaria efforts. In FY2008, Congress significantly increased its funding for global malaria and authorized the creation of the U.S. Global Malaria Coordinator at the United States Agency for International Development (USAID) to oversee all U.S. malaria efforts. President Barack Obama has also emphasized combating malaria in his Global Health Initiative (GHI). This report provides background information on malaria and explains the key components of the U.S. response.

DESCRIPTION OF MALARIA

Malaria is an infectious disease that is transmitted to people through the bite of infected mosquitoes. The disease infects red blood cells, causing a range of symptoms that include fever, headache, and vomiting. Although malaria is preventable and curable, if left untreated, it can be fatal. Young children, pregnant women, and individuals with HIV/AIDS are particularly vulnerable to malaria due to their weakened immune systems.

GLOBAL MALARIA STATISTICS[1]

Malaria Cases: The World Health Organization (WHO) estimates that half of the world's population is at risk of malaria infection. Malaria is prevalent in 106 countries, referred to as malaria-endemic countries. In 2010, there were approximately 216 million cases of malaria worldwide, down from approximately 233 million cases in 2000. Since 2000, 43 countries have reported a reduction in reported malaria cases of more than 50%. Likewise, the estimated incidence—new cases of malaria—has decreased by 17% globally between 2000 and 2010. Malaria Deaths: The malaria death toll declined from 985,000 in 2000 to 655,000 people in 2010. Roughly 86% of 2010 malaria-related deaths occurred among children younger than five. Since 2000, global malaria mortality has been reduced by 26%.

REGIONAL DISTRIBUTION OF MALARIA[2]

Malaria occurs worldwide, though it is heavily concentrated in what are categorized by WHO as the African, South-East Asian, and the Eastern Mediterranean regions (*Figure 1*).[3]

- In 2010, about 81% of all malaria cases and 91% of all malaria-related deaths occurred in the WHO Africa region. There are 43 malaria-endemic countries in the Africa region.
- The WHO Southeast Asia region was home to 13% of all malaria cases and 6% of malaria-related deaths in 2010. Of the 10 malaria-endemic countries in the South-East Asia region, India, Myanmar (Burma), and Indonesia make up 94% of all confirmed malaria cases.
- The WHO Eastern Mediterranean region was home to 5% of all malaria cases and 3% of malaria-related deaths in 2010. In the region, Sudan, Pakistan, Yemen, and Afghanistan make up 97% of confirmed malaria cases.

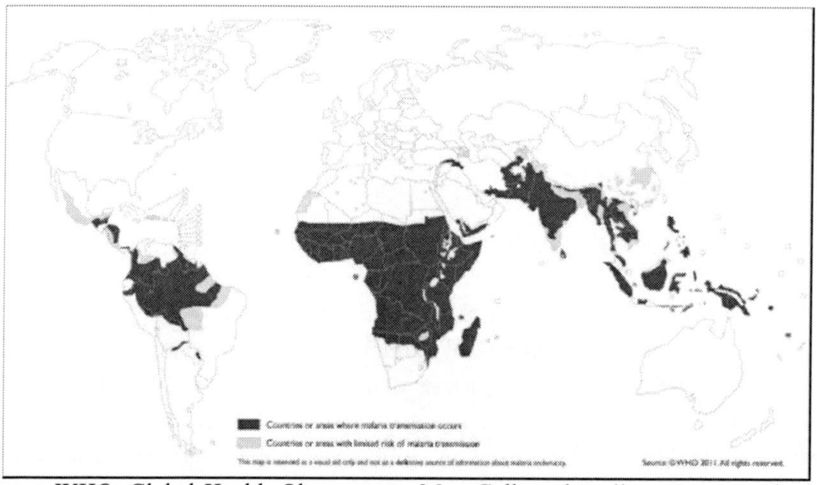

Source: WHO, Global Health Observatory, Map Gallery, http://gamapserver.who.int/mapLibrary/.

Notes: Countries or areas in dark blue are where malaria transmission occurs. Countries or areas in light blue are those with limited risk of malaria transmission.

Figure 1. Malaria, Countries or Areas at Risk of Transmission, 2010.

Malaria Prevention and Treatment

The international community generally applies four strategies for combating malaria:

Treatment: Anti-malarial treatments include chloroquine, primaquine, and artesmisinin-based combination therapy (ACT). ACT is the preferred treatment in areas with particularly deadly forms of malaria or with drug resistance to earlier generations of anti-malarials. Multi-drug resistant malaria is found worldwide, and there is evidence that ACT resistance is occurring in Asia.

Intermittent Preventive Treatment in Pregnancy (IPTp): In areas with high concentrations of malaria, physicians give pregnant women an anti-malarial drug to prevent them from transmitting the disease to their infants.

Insecticide-Treated Bed Nets (ITNs): Insecticides used to treat bed nets kill and repel mosquitoes. ITNs are used as personal protection against mosquito bites, but evidence suggests that high community coverage of ITNs can lower the number of mosquitoes in a general area and reduce the life span of mosquitoes that remain. ITNs retain cffective levels of insecticide for up to six months. Newly developed long-lasting insecticide-treated nets (LLINs) last for at least three years.

Indoor Residual Spraying (IRS): IRS involves covering household walls with an insecticide to kill any mosquito that comes into contact with the surfaces for several months. To be effective, IRS must be applied to a high percentage (80%) of household surfaces. Resistance to insecticides is a growing concern.

While there is presently no malaria vaccine, research is ongoing. There are currently over a dozen vaccine candidates in clinical development, and one, produced by GlaxoSmithKline, is in clinical trials.

KEY U.S. LEGISLATION ON GLOBAL MALARIA

- On December 27, 2000, President Bill Clinton signed into law the Assistance for International Malaria Control Act (P.L. 106-570). The act authorized $50 million per year for FY2001 and FY2002 for anti-malaria activities in countries with high malaria prevalence.
- On May 27, 2003, President George W. Bush signed into law the United States Leadership Against HIV/AIDS, Tuberculosis, and Malaria Act of 2003 (Leadership Act, P.L. 108-25). The act authorized $15 billion for global HIV/AIDS, TB, and malaria programs from FY2004 through FY2008. The act recognized malaria control as a major foreign policy objective, though it did not specify an amount for bilateral malaria programs. The act also prohibited U.S. contributions to the Global Fund to Fight AIDS, Tuberculosis and

Malaria (Global Fund) (see "Key Partners in the Response to Global Malaria") from exceeding 33% of funds contributed from all sources.

- On July 24, 2008, President Bush signed into law the Tom Lantos and Henry J. Hyde U.S. Global Leadership Against HIV/AIDS, Tuberculosis, and Malaria Reauthorization Act of 2008 (Lantos-Hyde Act, P.L. 110-293). The act authorized $48 billion for global HIV/AIDS, TB, and malaria programs from FY2008 through FY2013, including $5 billion for malaria programs over five years. The act also created the position of U.S. Global Malaria Coordinator at USAID. The Malaria Coordinator is charged with overseeing all U.S. anti-malaria efforts, submitting an annual report to Congress describing U.S. malaria programs, and developing a five-year strategic plan for U.S. efforts to combat malaria.

This legislation will be up for reauthorization in FY2013.

U.S. Global Malaria Programs

The United States has supported global malaria control efforts since the 1950s. Efforts to expand U.S. malaria programs and improve their coordination increased following the announcement of the President's Malaria Initiative (PMI) in 2005. PMI represented a growing acknowledgement of the efficacy of malaria prevention and treatment strategies and built on the success of the President's Emergency Plan for AIDS Relief (PEPFAR) in harnessing resources to combat a disease. PMI was initially created as a five-year, $1.2 billion effort to increase U.S. engagement in global malaria control and reduce malaria-related deaths by 50% in 15 high-burden focus countries. Focus countries were selected according to several criteria, including high malaria burden, capacity to implement anti-malaria programs, and willingness to partner with the United States. PMI has since expanded into four other malaria-endemic countries in Africa (*Table 1*).

PMI is an interagency initiative run by USAID and jointly implemented by USAID and the Centers for Disease Control and Prevention (CDC). The U.S. Global Malaria Coordinator at USAID coordinates malaria efforts across a number of agencies and departments, including CDC, the Department of Defense (DOD), and the National Institutes of Health (NIH). Oversight duties are shared with an Interagency Steering Group composed of representatives from USAID, CDC/the Department of Health and Human Services (HHS), the

Department of State, DOD, the National Security Council, and the Office of Management and Budget. USAID and CDC also provide bilateral malaria assistance to a handful of countries not designated as PMI focus countries.

Table 1. PMI Focus Countries

The PMI Focus Countries have been added over the course of several fiscal years:
FY2006: Angola, Tanzania, Uganda FY2007: Malawi, Mozambique, Rwanda, Senegal FY2008: Benin, Ethiopia, Ghana, Kenya, Liberia, Madagascar, Mali, Zambia FY2011: Nigeria, Democratic Republic of the Congo FY2012: Guinea and Zimbabwe

Note: PMI countries selected in FY2006, FY2007, and FY2008 represent the original 15 PMI focus countries.

President Obama has indicated support for an expanded U.S. malaria program. On May 5, 2009, the President announced Global Health Initiative (GHI), a new effort to develop a comprehensive U.S. global health strategy over the course of six years.

Malaria is one of the GHI's six priority areas, and PMI is considered a key component of the GHI, reflecting the Administration's belief that scaled-up malaria interventions can help maximize health impact per dollar spent. The GHI calls for a more integrated U.S. response to global health issues, including better coordination between malaria and maternal and child health programs.

The GHI also calls for a shift in U.S. global health strategy from one focused on specific diseases to a more comprehensive approach to health, including a focus on health system strengthening.

In April 2010, in response to congressional reporting requirements to develop a coordinated approach to global malaria, USAID, HHS (including CDC), and the Department of State released a joint "Lantos-Hyde United States Government Malaria Strategy."[4] The strategy explains how U.S. malaria programs will advance the goals of the GHI and outlines key targets for the U.S. malaria program from 2009 to 2014. Key goals include the following:

- halve the burden of malaria (morbidity and mortality) in 70% of at-risk populations in sub-Saharan Africa;
- limit the spread of anti-malarial multi-drug resistance in Southeast Asia and the Americas;
- assist host countries to revise and update their National Malaria Control Strategies and Plans to reflect the declining burden of malaria; and
- link U.S. malaria efforts with host country malaria plans.

IMPLEMENTING U.S. AGENCIES

U.S. agencies supporting global malaria control efforts include the following:

- *United States Agency for International Development*: USAID manages PMI programs in the PMI focus countries. USAID also supports malaria control programs in several other countries and facilitates efforts to identify and contain anti-malarial drug resistance through two regional programs in the Amazon Basin and the Mekong Delta. USAID's malaria programs focus on five key areas: IRS, ITNs, IPTp, diagnosis and treatment, and pesticide management.
- *Centers for Disease Control and Prevention:* CDC jointly implements PMI with USAID. CDC's malaria efforts focus on monitoring and evaluation, disease surveillance, and capacity development for national malaria control programs. CDC also undertakes global malaria research to improve prevention and treatment efforts with an emphasis on LLINs, IRS, and IPTp, and the elimination of malaria.
- *Department of Defense:* DOD supports malaria research, including anti-malaria treatment and vaccine development. Research is conducted at the U.S. Military Malaria Vaccine Program at the Walter Reed Army Institute of Research and the Malaria Research Department at the Navy Medical Research Center.
- *National Institutes of Health:* The National Institute of Allergy and Infectious Diseases (NIAID) of the NIH is the lead U.S. agency supporting malaria research. NIAID works on developing tools for malaria prevention, treatment, and control, and enhancing research infrastructure in malaria-endemic countries.

U.S. Global Malaria Assistance Funds

Congress designates funds for malaria to USAID, through State-Foreign Operations appropriations, and to CDC, through Labor, Health and Human Services, and Education appropriations. Congress also provides resources to the DOD and NIH for malaria research efforts. Congressional appropriations for malaria have consistently increased since FY2004. In response to growing calls within the international community for global malaria control, funding for malaria interventions has increased most precipitously since FY2007 (*Table 2* and *Figure 2*) in support of PMI expansion into new countries.

Table 2. U.S. Bilateral Funding for Malaria: FY2004-FY2013 ($ millions, current)

Program /Agency	FY 2004 Actual	FY 2005 Actual	FY 2006 Actual	FY 2007 Actual	FY 2008 Actual	FY 2009 Actual	FY 2010 Actual	FY 2011 Actual	FY 2012 Estimate	FY 2013 Request
USAID GHP[a]	79.6	79.4	98.9	248.0	347.2	382.5	585.0	618.8	650.0	619.0
USAID Other[b]	0.0	0.0	0.0	0.0	2.4	2.5	0.0	0.0	0.0	0.0
CDC	9.2	9.1	9.0	8.9	8.7	9.4	9.4	9.2	9.2	9.4
NIH	88.6	103.8	98.0	111.8	132.5	121.0	112.0	145.0	147.0	147.0
DOD	21.0	22.0	18.0	29.0	31.0	30.6	26.4	27.4	0.0	0.0
TOTAL Malaria Bilateral	198.4	214.3	223.9	397.7	521.8	546.8	732.8	800.3	806.2	775.4

Source: Compiled by CRS from Congressional Budget Justifications, appropriations legislation, and PMI reports.

[a]Global Health Programs (GHP) Account.

[b] This includes funding from the Development Assistance Account (DA), the Economic Support Fund Account (ESF), and the Assistance for Europe, Eurasia, and Central Asia Account (AEECA).

The United States also supports global malaria programs through contributions to the Global Fund, an international financing mechanism for the response to HIV/AIDS, TB, and malaria. U.S. contributions to the Global Fund support grants for HIV/AIDS, TB, and malaria. The United States is the single largest donor to the Global Fund. *Table 3* details U.S. contributions to the Global Fund from FY2004 to FY2013.

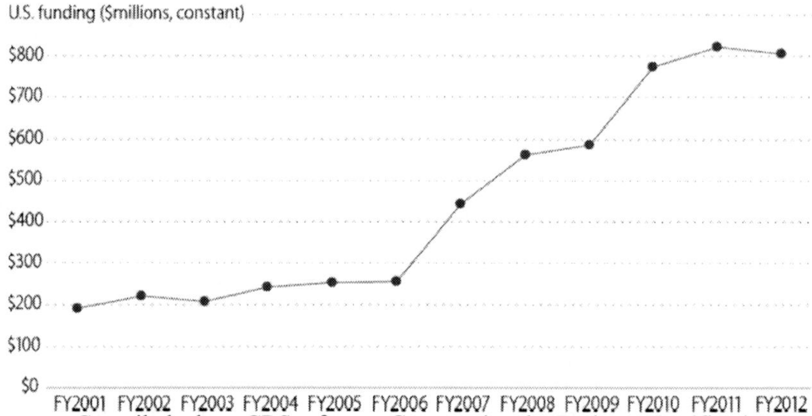

Source: Compiled by CRS from Congressional Budget Justifications and appropriations legislation.

Figure 2. U.S. Bilateral Funding for Malaria in Constant Dollars: FY2001-FY2012. ($ millions, constant)

Table 3. U.S.Appropriations for the Global Fund: FY2004-FY2013 ($ millions, current)

Program /Agency	FY 2004 Actual	FY 2005 Actual	FY 2006 Actual	FY 2007 Actual	FY 2008 Actual	FY 2009 Actual	FY 2010 Actual	FY 2011 Actual	FY 2012 Esti-mate	FY 2013 Request
USAID	397.6	248.0	247.5	247.5	0.0	100.0	0.0	0.0	0.0	0.0
State	0.0	0.0	198.0	377.5	545.5	600.0	750.0	748.5	1,300.0	1,650.0
HHS	149.1	99.2	99.0	99.0	294.8	300.0	300.0	297.3	0.0	0.0
Total	546.6	347.2	544.5	724.0	840.3	1,000.0	1,050.0	1,045.8	1,300.0	1,650.0

Source: Compiled by CRS from Congressional Budget Justifications and appropriations legislation.

The majority of total global funding for malaria control comes from three sources: external donor assistance, national government spending, and household expenditures. According to WHO, of the total malaria spending in 2007, donor assistance accounted for 47%, national government spending accounted for 34%, and household expenditures accounted for 19%.[5] The Global Fund is the single largest donor for global malaria efforts. WHO estimates that in 2010, the Global Fund accounted for approximately 50% of malaria funds from international sources, while PMI, DFID, and the World

Bank accounted for approximately 49% of international funding (*Figure 3*). International disbursements for global malaria appear to have peaked in 2011.[6]

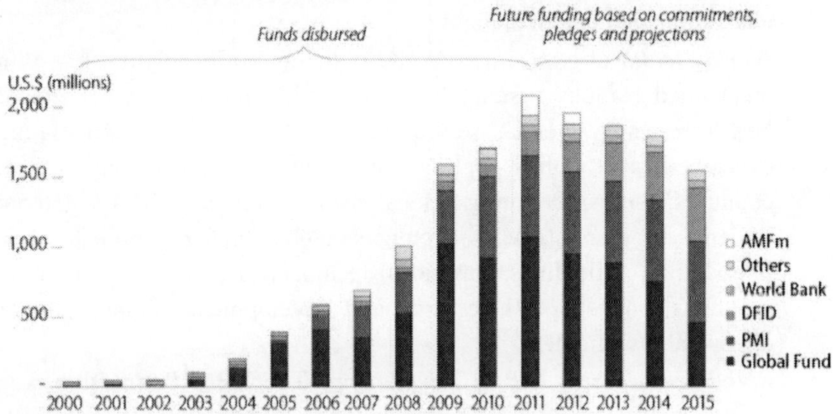

Source: Data from WHO, World Malaria Report, 2011, p. 15.

Figure 3. Past and Projected International Funding for Malaria Control, 2000-2015.

KEY PARTNERS IN THE RESPONSE TO GLOBAL MALARIA

The United States works with a range of partners to combat malaria, including other national governments, multilateral organizations, non-governmental organizations (NGOs), and the private sector. Key partners include the following:

- *The Global Fund:* The Global Fund was established in 2002 as a public-private partnership to provide significant financial support for the global response to HIV/AIDS, TB, and malaria. The United States contributes more to the Global Fund than any other donor. The Global Fund has committed over $22.6 billion in grants in 150 countries since it was established and provides over half of all international funding for malaria control in endemic countries.[7] In November 2011, the Global Fund announced that due to limited resources available, it would postpone its 11th round of funding.[8]
- *The World Bank:* In 2005, the World Bank launched the World Bank Booster Program for Malaria Control in Africa. The Booster Program

is implemented in 18 countries and supports the rapid scale-up of preexisting malaria control interventions and works to strengthen in-country procurement and supply-chain capacity, monitoring, and evaluation, and health planning.

- *World Health Organization:* WHO is the authority for health within the United Nations system. It is responsible for shaping the global health research agenda, setting norms and standards, articulating evidence-based policy options, providing technical support to countries, and monitoring global health trends. WHO's Global Malaria Program (GMP) promotes global malaria policies and intervention guidelines, provides technical assistance to malaria programs, and supports research and development of anti-malarial drugs and insecticides.
- *Roll Back Malaria (RBM) Partnership:* The RBM Partnership was created in 1998 by WHO, United Nations Children's Fund (UNICEF), United Nations Development Program (UNDP), and the World Bank to facilitate coordination of malaria activities and optimal use of resources. The RBM Partnership has 500 partners, including malaria-endemic countries, Organization for Economic Cooperation and Development (OECD) donor governments, multilateral organizations, the private sector, NGOs, foundations, research institutions, and ex-officio members. The Coordinator of PMI currently sits on the RBM Partnership Board.
- *United Nations Children's Fund (UNICEF):* UNICEF supports malaria programs through its work on child survival and development. UNICEF assists in developing national malaria plans and policies; monitoring and evaluation; and supplying, procuring, and distributing malaria commodities. According to UNICEF, it is the world's largest procurer and deliverer of ITNs.[9] UNICEF and USAID have a "Malaria Control Partnership" to support malaria programming and commodity procurement, supply, and distribution.
- *American Red Cross:* The American Red Cross malaria programs support distribution of ITNs, community education on the threat of malaria and the proper use of ITNs, and operational research on the effectiveness of ITNs.
- *Bill and Melinda Gates Foundation:* The Gates Foundation advocates increased support for malaria and funds the development of new tools to treat, diagnose, and prevent malaria. The foundation hopes to have supported the development of a malaria vaccine by 2025.[10]

KEY ISSUES IN GLOBAL MALARIA

The 112th Congress will likely be faced with a number of issues regarding the U.S. response to global malaria, including how much assistance to provide and how to best apportion global malaria funds. Over the past decade, significant progress has been made in combating global malaria. International assistance has helped to lower the number of malaria cases and deaths around the world. At the same time, several key challenges threaten the progress achieved to date. As Congress continues to debate the role of the United States in global malaria control, it might consider the following issues:

- *Insecticide and drug resistance:* Growing instances of drug-resistant malaria and insecticide-resistant mosquitoes threaten global malaria control, particularly in Southeast Asia and Africa. There are currently no alternatives to available forms of insecticides and treatments. Some health experts argue that anti-malaria resources should prioritize drug and insecticide resistance, including efforts to improve drug quality control, resistance monitoring and surveillance, and research and development of new forms of malaria drugs.
- *Health System Strengthening:* Weak health systems have been a major impediment to successful malaria prevention and treatment. In particular, shortages in health care personnel and weak supply chain networks have limited the delivery of essential commodities for malaria control. There is some disagreement within the global health community about whether PMI has had a beneficial or detrimental impact on the broader functioning of health systems.
- *Control vs. elimination:* There is debate within the global health community over the degree to which the international community should commit itself to malaria control (reducing the disease burden to a level at which it is no longer a public health problem) or malaria elimination (reducing incidence of infection to zero in a defined geographic). While the majority of international funding for malaria efforts in the past decade has been focused on control efforts, a number of experts have argued that efforts should increasingly focus on elimination of the disease. Key issues affecting the debate over control versus elimination include whether countries have the capacity to support more ambitious programs, whether donor assistance is predictable enough to support elimination efforts, and how the

international community can avoid any potentially detrimental consequences of an elimination campaign, such as increased insecticide and drug resistance.

End Notes

[1] All data in this section is from World Health Organization (WHO), Global Malaria Program, World Malaria Report, 2011, http://www.who.int/malaria/world_malaria_report_2011/ 9789241564403_eng.pdf.

[2] All data in this section is from WHO, Global Malaria Program, World Malaria Report, 2011.

[3] For an explanation of the countries included in each WHO Region, see "WHO Regional Offices," http://www.who.int/about/regions/en/index.html.

[4] USAID, HHS, CDC, and Department of State, Lantos-Hyde United States Government Malaria Strategy: 2009-2014, April 25, 2010, http://www.fightingmalaria.gov/resources/reports/ usg_strategy2009-2014.pdf.

[5] WHO, World Malaria Report, 2009, p. 57, http://whqlibdoc.who.int/publications/2009/9789 241563901_eng.pdf.

[6] WHO, World Malaria Report, 2011, p. 15, http://www.who.int/ malaria/world_ malaria_ report_2011/ 9789241564403_eng.pdf.

[7] Global Fund to Fight AIDS, Tuberculosis, and Malaria, Making a Difference – Global Fund Results Report 2011, 2011, p. 42.

[8] The Global Fund to Fight AIDS, Tuberculosis, and Malaria, "The Global Fund is Alive and Well, but Global Health Progress is in Peril," December 2011, http://www.theglobalfund. org/en/mediacenter/announcements/2011-12- 01_The_Global_Fund_is_alive /.

[9] UNICEF website, "UNICEF in Action: Malaria," http://www.unicef.org/health/index_ malaria.html.

[10] Bill and Melinda Gates Foundation website, "Malaria: Our Approach," http://www.gates foundation.org/topics/Pages/ malaria.aspx#.

In: United States' Global Health Assistance
Editors: Kurk B. Weller
ISBN: 978-1-62948-387-0

Chapter 5

PROGRESS IN COMBATING NEGLECTED TROPICAL DISEASES (NTDS): U.S. AND GLOBAL EFFORTS FROM FY2006 TO FY2013*

Tiaji Salaam-Blyther

SUMMARY

The term "neglected tropical diseases" (NTDs) was coined by the World Health Organization (WHO) in 2003 to describe a set of diseases that are ancient, worsen poverty, and typically impair health and productivity while carrying low death rates. Some NTDs are easily treatable; others are not.

While the use of the term "NTDs" has helped to raise awareness about these longstanding health challenges, its use risks simplifying a complicated health challenge. Health interventions to address the array of NTDs vary, but a common factor to an enduring solution to these illnesses is economic development. Industrialized countries, including the United States, have controlled these diseases in their territories by combining drug treatment with the construction and use of improved sanitation, modernization of agricultural practices, and utilization of

---

* This is an edited, reformatted and augmented version of a Congressional Research Service publication, CRS Report for Congress R42931, from www.crs.gov, prepared for Members and Committees of Congress, dated January 22, 2013.

improved water systems. Neglected tropical diseases are diseases that primarily plague the poorest people in developing countries. Changes in the environment and population flows, however, make industrialized countries, including the United States, increasingly vulnerable to some NTDs, particularly dengue haemorrhagic fever, for which there is no cure.

Congressional interest in NTDs has been growing. Appropriations for NTD programs have steadily increased from $15 million in FY2006 to $89 million in FY2012. The Administration requested $67 million to support NTD programs in FY2013. In addition to raising spending for NTDs, Congress has taken other actions to demonstrate support for tackling NTDs. In October 2009, for example, the House Malaria Caucus expanded its purview to include NTDs. The Senate Malaria Caucus did the same in September 2012.

The international community has made substantial progress in combating select NTDs, though some have been tackled more effectively than others. Guinea worm disease, for example, is on the cusp of eradication.

More generally, expanding access to mass drug administration is contributing to decreases in prevalence of several NTDs, particularly across Latin America. Despite these advances, WHO cautions that these diseases cannot be banished without improving global access to clean water and sanitation, strengthening local health capacity (veterinary as well as human), and intensifying case detection and management. Making improvements in these areas will require long-term investments that are complex and may entail facing thorny issues such as addressing corruption, transferring ownership of health programs from donors to recipient countries, and evaluating the impact of political and economic policies on health programs (e.g., international lending requirements).

The United States has played an important role in combating NTDs, and President Barack Obama has prioritized tackling NTDs. Recommendations for congressional action may largely reflect broader arguments about congressional engagement in improving global health. Analysts who support congressional directives that set programmatic targets, outline the types of activities to be implemented in U.S. global health programs, and mandate reporting requirements would probably argue for the 113th Congress to take similar steps. Observers who maintain that these steps make U.S. global health programs less effective by minimizing the capacity of implementing agencies to adapt global health programs to local conditions would likely argue for limiting congressional support for combating NTDs to appropriating sufficient resources. This report discusses the prevalence of NTDs, U.S. and global actions to address them, and options the 113th Congress might consider.

INTRODUCTION

Over the past decade, global health has become a priority in U.S. foreign policy, and U.S. appropriations for global health-related efforts have more than tripled. Neglected tropical diseases (NTDs) have become an important part of these efforts.[1] Congressional appropriations for NTDs have grown from $15 million in FY2006 to $89 million in FY2012. The Administration requested $67 million to support NTD programs in FY2013. Heightened congressional interest in combating NTDs has been reflected not only in higher appropriation levels but also in the development of caucuses on these issues. In October 2009, the House Malaria Caucus expanded its purview to include NTDs, and in September 2012, the Senate Malaria Caucus did the same.

Tropical diseases encompass all diseases that occur solely, or principally, in the tropics.[2] Of these, the World Health Organization (WHO) describes 17 as "neglected tropical diseases," as until recently, resources for curing, controlling, and researching improved treatments for these were limited. The 17 NTDs are found mostly among the poorest people in 149 countries and territories (*Figure 1*), primarily where access to clean water, sanitation, and health services is limited. Some NTDs are transmitted by people; others are spread by vectors like snails, flies, or mosquitoes; and several others proliferate in contaminated sources (like infested soil or water). Among the 17 NTDs, 7 account for roughly 90% of the global NTD burden (*Table 1*). These are the three soil-transmitted helminthiases [intestinal worms (STH)], schistosomiasis (snail fever), lymphatic filariasis (elephantiasis), trachoma, and onchocerciasis (river blindness). Intestinal worms or STH account for more than 80% of the seven most common NTDs (*Figure 2*).

Drugs used in global NTD programs to treat the seven most common NTDs are donated or sold by pharmaceutical companies at subsidized prices ranging between $0.02 and $2.23 per dose. These drugs are taken once or twice annually.[3] Although costs vary by location, treating these diseases has become increasingly inexpensive relative to other diseases that commonly afflict the poor in developing countries (*Table 2*). The cost of treating some NTDs has dropped in part because medicines to treat several of the most common NTDs are interchangeable and can be used to treat more than one disease. In addition, treatments for the most common NTDs can be dispensed to a broad population irrespective of individual disease status. This process, known as mass drug administration (MDA), has become an important tool in global efforts to control and eliminate NTDs.

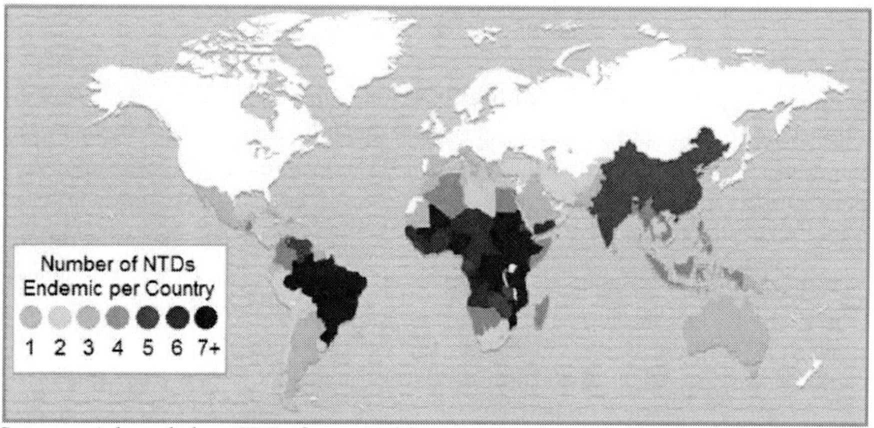

Source: Adapted by CRS from Uniting to Combat NTDs, http://www.unitingtocombatntds.org/downloads/press/ntd_event_burden_map_updated.pdf, accessed on October 25, 2012.

Figure 1. Global NTD Burden Map.

Table 1. 17 Neglected Tropical Diseases

Seven Most Common NTDs (90% of all NTDs)	Other NTDs
Lymphatic Filariasis (Elephantiasis)	Buruli Ulcer
Onchocerciasis (River Blindness)	Chagas Disease
Schistosomiasis (Snail Fever)	Cysticercosis/Taeniasis
Soil-Transmitted Helminthiases (STH)	Dengue
• Hookworm	Dracunculiasis (Guinea worm disease)
• Whipworm	Echinococcosis
• Roundworm	Foodborne Trematode Infections
Trachoma	Human African Trypanosomiasis (Sleeping Sickness)
	Leishmaniasis
	Leprosy
	Rabies
	Yaws

Source: Created by CRS from WHO website on NTDs, http://www.who.int/neglected_diseases/diseases/en/, accessed on November 7, 2012.

Table 2. Annual Per Patient Cost of Treating Key Infectious Diseases Globally (U.S. dollars)

Disease	Low Estimate	High Estimate
HIV/AIDS	100.00	335.00
Tuberculosis	100.00	500.00
Malaria	0.50	1.40
NTDs	0.02	2.23

Sources: HIV/AIDS data was compiled from UNAIDS, World AIDS Day Report, 2012, p. 17 and Department of State, The President's Emergency Plan for AIDS Relief Eighth Annual Report to Congress, 2012, p. 3. Tuberculosis data was taken from WHO, Global Tuberculosis Report, 2012, p. 52. Malaria data was taken from WHO, World Malaria Report, 2011, p. x,. NTD data was taken from WHO, Accelerating Work to Overcome the Global Impact of Neglected Tropical Diseases: A Roadmap for Implementation, 2012, p. 16.

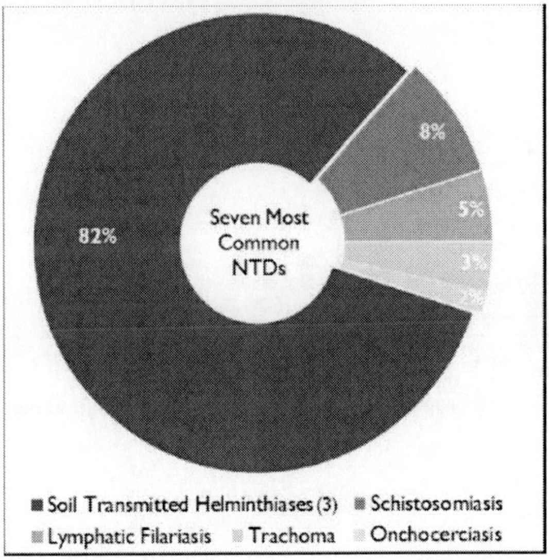

Source: Created by CRS from Peter Hotez, Forgotten People, Forgotten Diseases (Washington, DC: ASM Press, 2008).

Figure 2. Estimated Prevalence of Seven Most Common NTDs.

GLOBAL PROGRESS IN COMBATING NTDS

Tremendous progress has been made in tackling NTDs since 2003, when the term "neglected tropical diseases" was coined at the first WHO meeting on a set of diseases that worsened poverty and for which solutions had not been prioritized. Until then, the international community had emphasized some of these diseases, but interventions for others languished. Two diseases for which long-term international focus has led to considerable reductions in incidence are dracunculiasis (Guinea worm disease), which has been nearly eradicated, and sleeping sickness, whose cases have dropped by some 75%. Since 1986, the number of new Guinea worm disease cases has fallen by 99% (*Figure 3*). By the end of 2011, the disease was endemic in only four countries: Chad, Ethiopia, Mali, and South Sudan. Nearly 97% of the 1,058 cases identified in 2011 occurred in South Sudan, where instability remains a key threat to eradication.

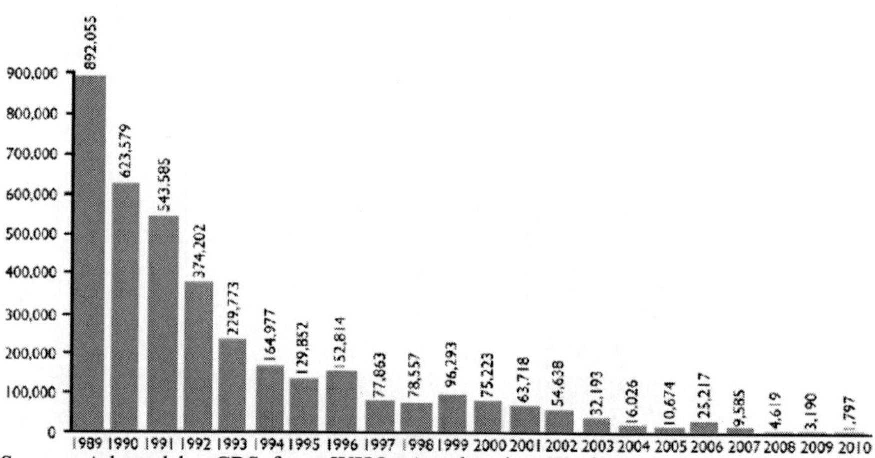

Source: Adapted by CRS from WHO, Accelerating Work to Overcome the Global Impact of Neglected Tropical Diseases: A Roadmap for Implementation, 2012, p. 10.

Figure 3. Global Guinea Worm Disease Cases: 1989-2010.

Important advances have been seen as well in decreasing new cases of Human African Trypanosomiasis (sleeping sickness). After seeing increases in annual cases over a decade, reports of new sleeping sickness cases began to drop precipitously in 1999. From 1998 through 2010, reported cases fell by roughly 75% (*Figure 4*).

Progress in tackling NTDs is rooted in several factors:

- large, open-ended donations by pharmaceutical companies;
- increased funding from donors;

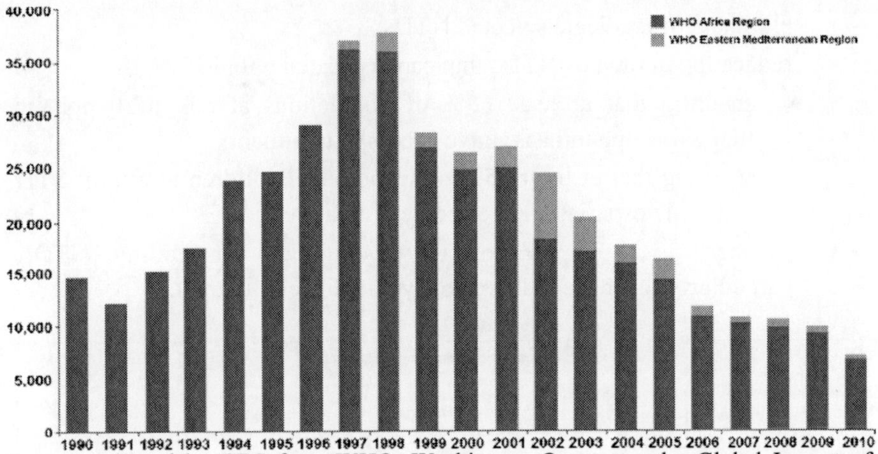

Source: Adapted by CRS from WHO, Working to Overcome the Global Impact of Neglected Tropical Diseases: Update 2011, 2011, p. 7.

Figure 4. Global Sleeping Sickness Cases: 1990-2010.

- intensified attention by the international community;
- integrated disease treatment regimens; and
- enhanced cooperation among recipient countries, pharmaceutical companies, non-governmental organizations (NGOs), and donors.

Countries develop national NTD plans and receive financial support from donors to implement them. The WHO and donors, such as the U.S. Agency for International Development (USAID), review drug donation applications and support country-level planning, training, and monitoring and evaluation. Drug companies provide treatments used for national NTD plans, either for free or at highly discounted rates. NGOs and faith-based organizations partner with recipient countries to implement the NTD plans. Academic groups, public-private partnerships, and pharmaceutical companies research and develop innovative treatments and control mechanisms.

Global Actions in 2012

In 2007, WHO released the *Global Plan to Combat Neglected Tropical Diseases*, which outlined several goals and targets for global control, elimination, and eradication of NTDs by 2015.[4] Three key goals included in the plan were to

- eliminate or eradicate selected NTDs;
- reduce the burden of NTDs that can be treated with MDA[5] by:
  - ensuring that at least 65% of populations at risk of lymphatic filariasis (elphantiasis) have access to treatment;
  - ensuring that at least 75% of school-aged children at risk of STH and schistosomiasis have access to treatment;
- advance novel approaches to treating and controlling NTDs, particularly for those that are costly and difficult to treat.

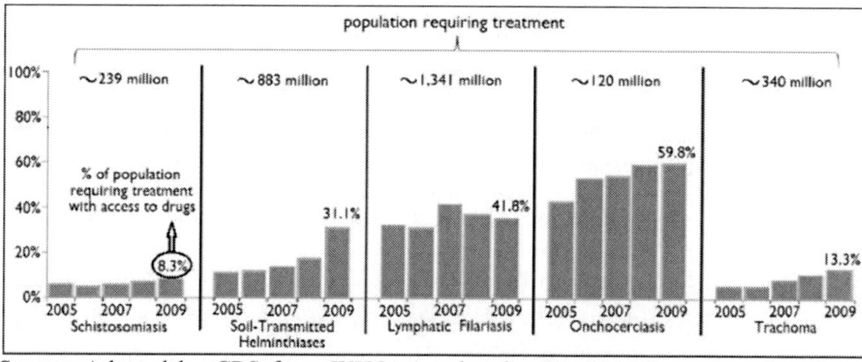

Source: Adapted by CRS from WHO, Accelerating Work to Overcome the Global Impact of Neglected Tropical Diseases: A Roadmap for Implementation, 2012, p. 6.

Figure 5. Global Access to Drugs for Seven Most Common NTDs: 2005-2009.

In 2012, WHO released a report that highlighted progress in reaching the 2015 goals and set new ones for 2020.[6] Key goals include

- ensuring supply of drugs and other interventions to help:
  - *eradicate* Guinea worm disease.
  - *eliminate* elephantiasis, leprosy, sleeping sickness, and blinding trachoma by 2020.
  - *control* snail fever, soil-transmitted helminthiases (STH), Chagas disease, visceral leishmaniasis, and river blindness by 2020;[7]
- advancing R&D to identify next-generation treatments and interventions; and
- providing technical support, tools, and resources for monitoring and evaluation.

The report noted progress in treating onchocerciasis (river blindness), but little improvement in expanding access to medicines for schistosomiasis (snail fever) and soil-transmitted helminthiases due to inadequate drug supply (*Figure 5*). Insufficient progress in tackling STH is important, as these diseases account for roughly 80% of the seven most common NTDs (*Figure 2*).

The London Declaration on Neglected Tropical Diseases

Following the release of the 2012 WHO report, 13 pharmaceutical companies, the Bill & Melinda Gates Foundation (Gates Foundation), the World Bank, several NGOs, and officials representing the United States, Britain, and the United Arab Emirates (UAE) convened in London, England, to reaffirm their commitment to combatting NTDs. Participants signed the *London Declaration on Neglected Tropical Diseases*, which highlighted the role each signatory would play in reaching the 2020 goals outlined in the WHO report.

Implementing partners agreed to donate a range of treatments, funds, intellectual property rights, and research and development (R&D) resources. *Appendix A* lists the funding commitments and activities donors pledged to support.[8] These pledges included

- $785 million (includes pre-existing commitments) to strengthen drug distribution and program implementation;
- 1.4 billion drug treatments annually;
- access to drug compound libraries to identify new treatments;
- increased financial support for NTD programs (some of which amended previous commitments to ongoing efforts), such as:
  - a five-year, $363 million pledge by the Gates Foundation,
  - a five-year, £245 million (roughly $393 million) pledge by Britain, and
  - a joint $40 million donation to the Carter Center by UAE, Gates Foundation, and the Children's Investment Fund Foundation;
- commitments by the governments of Bangladesh, Brazil, Mozambique, and Tanzania to devote political and financial resources to combat endemic NTDs.

Pledges by pharmaceutical companies to support research and development (R&D) on new treatments, vaccines, and testing supplies is vital considering the emergence of evidence that hookworm, one of the STHs (that comprise 80% of all NTDs), may be developing resistance to existing medication.[9] Concerns about drug resistance aside, R&D commitments are also important as signatories of the London Declaration indicate existing tools are not sufficient to meet the WHO 2020 goals (*Figure 6*).

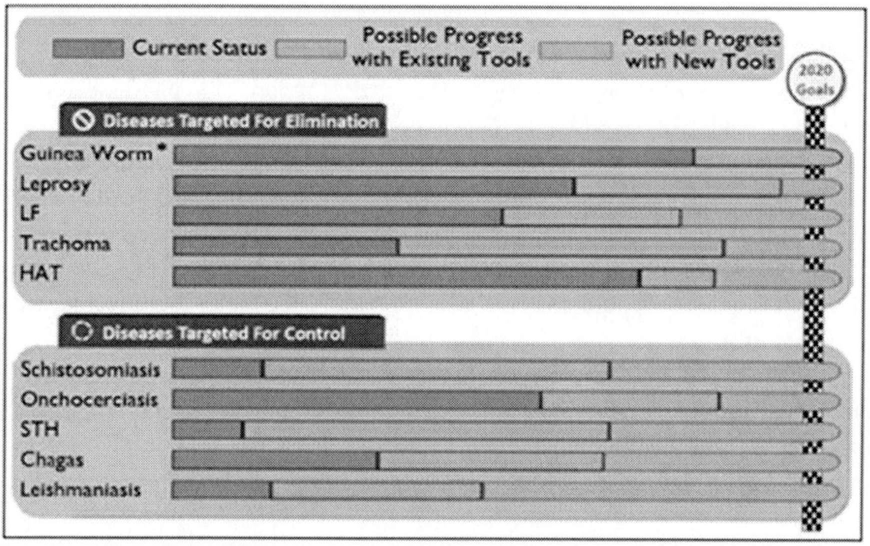

Source: Adapted by CRS from Uniting to Combat NTDs, http://www.unitingtocombatntds.org/downloads/ press/ntd_event_2020_goals_graphic.pdf, accessed on October 25, 2012.

Notes: "Possible progress with existing tools" predicts advancement of elimination and control efforts without development of new tools. "Possible progress with new tools" predicts advancements that could be made if new tools were developed, such as more effective treatments and vaccines.

* Guinea worm disease is targeted for eradication.

Acronyms: Lymphatic Filariasis (LF), Human African Trypanosomiasis (HAT), Soil-Transmitted Helminthiases (STH).

Figure 6. Global Progress on 2020 Goals.

U.S. EFFORTS TO TACKLE NTDS

U.S.-based institutions have long supported efforts to control NTDs. These institutions include the federal government, pharmaceutical companies, philanthropic organizations, and NGOs. Key U.S. government players include the U.S. Agency for International Development (USAID), U.S. Centers for Disease Control and Prevention (CDC), National Institutes of Health (NIH), and Department of Defense (DOD).[10] NGOs include groups like the Carter Center and RTI International; philanthropic organizations include the Gates Foundation and the Sabin Vaccine Institute; and private companies include Merck, Johnson & Johnson and Pfizer. While each of these plays an important role in combating NTDs, this section focuses exclusively on the USAID-managed NTD Program.[11]

In 2006, the Bush Administration launched the Neglected Tropical Disease Control Program, the first U.S. effort to address a group of NTDs. The program was created in response to language in the FY2006 Foreign Operations Appropriations Act, which made available up to $15 million "to support an integrated response to the control of neglected diseases including intestinal parasites [STH], schistosomiasis, lymphatic filariasis, onchocerciasis, trachoma and leprosy."[12] The language signaled congressional support for calls to integrate and expand access to drugs for the seven most common NTDs. Until that time, most countries and their implementing partners focused on tackling a single NTD. The NTD Program sought to document the feasibility of integrating treatment for several NTDs and advance application of this strategy. At the outset, the NTD program aimed to support the provision of 160 million NTD treatments to 40 million people in 15 countries. In 2008, President George W. Bush reaffirmed his commitment to the program and proposed spending $350 million over six years (from FY2008 through FY2013) on expanding the program to 30 countries.[13]

During his first term, President Barack Obama named the NTD Program a priority. While announcing the Global Health Initiative (GHI) in May 2009,[14] President Obama indicated the NTD Program would be a key part of the initiative and would be increasingly integrated into other global health efforts. The 2009-2014 Lantos-Hyde United States Government Malaria Strategy exemplifies this priority by outlining how the Administration plans to integrate malaria and NTD activities with other U.S. global health efforts.[15]

Through GHI, the Obama Administration seeks to

- administer 1 billion NTD treatments,
- halve the prevalence of the seven most common NTDs by 2013,
- eliminate leprosy in all endemic countries by 2016,
- eliminate onchocerciasis in Latin America by 2016, and
- eliminate lymphatic filariasis globally by 2017.

Through the first half of FY2012, the NTD Program had supported the provision of 584.6 million treatments (*Figure 7*) to 257.9 million people across 20 countries. A map of the countries is in *Appendix B*.

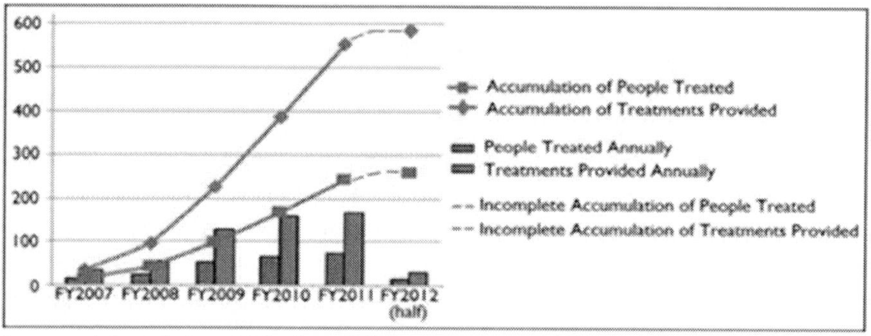

Source: Adapted by CRS from NTD Program website at http://www.neglecteddiseases.gov/about/index.html, accessed on November 28, 2012.

Figure 7. NTD Treatments Administered in USAID Programs: FY2007-FY2012.

FY2013 Funding

USAID has spent more than $300 million on the NTD Program since it began in FY2006 through FY2012 (*Figure 8*). The FY2013 budget request includes $67 million for the program. The 112th Congress did not complete legislation for FY2013 Foreign Operations Appropriations, through which the program is funded. The House Appropriations Committee included positive language about the program but did not specify an amount for the NTD effort in its committee report. The Senate Appropriations Committee recommended $125 million for the program in its committee report.

Issues for Congress

The international community has made substantial progress in combating select neglected tropical diseases. Some NTDs have been tackled more effectively than others. Guinea worm disease, for example, is on the cusp of eradication and with expanding mass drug administration campaigns, the prevalence of several NTDs is declining, particularly in Latin America. Despite these advancements, WHO cautions in the 2020 Roadmap that these diseases cannot be banished without improving global access to clean water and sanitation, strengthening local health capacity (veterinary as well as human), and intensifying case detection and management.

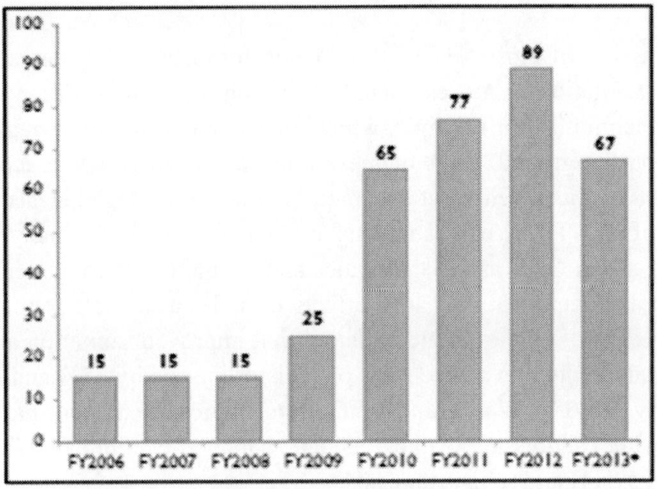

Source: Adapted by CRS from USAID website, http://www.neglecteddiseaess.gov/funding/index.html, accessed on October 25, 2012.

Notes: *FY2013 amount is a budgetary request.

Figure 8. USAID Spending on the NTD Program: FY2006-FY2012.(current U.S. $ millions).

The United States has played an important role in combating NTDs and will likely be a central player in global efforts to advance the 2020 NTD goals. Recommendations for congressional action may largely reflect broader arguments about the appropriate role for Congress in improving global health. Analysts who applaud congressional directives that set programmatic targets, outline the types of activities to be implemented in U.S. global health programs, and mandate reporting requirements would probably argue for the 113th Congress to take similar steps in meeting the 2020 NTD goals. Observers who maintain that these steps make U.S. global health programs less effective by minimizing the capacity of implementing agencies to adapt global health programs to local conditions would likely argue for limiting congressional support for combating NTDs to appropriating sufficient resources.

The section below discusses a range of issues U.S. and international organizations may face as they attempt to reach the WHO 2020 goals, as well as those set by the Administration (see “U.S. Efforts to Tackle NTDs”). Some of the discussion includes an analysis of steps the 113th Congress might consider.

Accessing Clean Water and Sanitation

Transmission of most NTDs is facilitated by insufficient access to clean water and sanitation.[16] An estimated 2 billion people are carrying soil-transmitted helminths, for example, which are spread primarily through openly defecating on the ground. Eggs of these intestinal worms, which account for roughly 80% of the seven most common NTDs (which together account for about 90% of all NTD cases), can persist in the environment for many years.

Experts at the CDC assert that water and sanitation improvement should be a central component of any effective and sustainable approach to controlling NTDs.[17] One estimate indicates that improved sanitation and water safety can reduce the prevalence rates of schistosomiasis by 75% and blinding trachoma by 25%.[18] Water and sanitation improvement are particularly important when addressing pathogens that cannot be eliminated by drugs alone, such as STH and schistosomiasis.

Several experts urge greater investments in water and sanitation and see attainment of global water and sanitation goals as an important step towards eliminating NTDs.[19] Through the Millennium Development Goals (MDGs), the international community sought to halve the share of people without access to clean water and basic sanitation by 2015.[20] WHO estimated that between 2005 and 2015, it would cost $72 billion annually to implement and maintain enough water and sanitation schemes to meet global water and sanitation targets, of which $54 billion would need to be spent on maintaining the systems.[21] In 2010, members of the Organization for Economic Cooperation and Development (OECD) committed $7.8 billion towards improving global access to clean drinking water and sanitation.[22] U.S. and global investments in sanitation would need to increase significantly to meet this funding gap.

The 113th Congress has at its disposal an important tool for ensuring U.S. water and sanitation resources are used to reinforce the NTD Program. The Senator Paul Simon Water for the Poor Act (P.L. 109-121), which amends the Foreign Assistance Act of 1961, requires the Secretary of State to develop a strategy for expanding global access to clean water and sanitation. The act specifies that the strategy should include specific and measurable goals, benchmarks, and timetables to achieve the objective described in [the strategy];

methods to coordinate and integrate United States water and sanitation assistance programs with other United States development assistance programs to achieve the objective described [in the strategy].[23]

As of the publication of this report, the Administration had not yet released a water strategy, though one is reportedly imminent.[24] The 113th Congress could request testimony from Administration officials on the progress in developing a strategy and integrating other development assistance programs, including global health programs like the NTD Program per legislation.

Integrating the U.S. NTD Program

Investments in water and sanitation are considered important, as mass drug administration campaigns cannot be used in isolation to eliminate NTDs. The process of combating diseases by combining responses by practitioners across sectors, particularly those related to health, agriculture, water, construction, and waste disposal, is known as integrated vector management. Indeed, the United States was unable to control hookworm (an STH) within its own borders until the early 1900s, when an integrated vector management (IVM) approach was applied.[25] WHO maintains that an effective NTD response would use an intersectoral approach that is based on five areas:

1. mass drug administration;
2. intensified case-management;
3. vector control;
4. safe water, sanitation, and hygiene; and
5. veterinary public health (by also controlling the NTDs that are zoonotic).[26]

It is unclear whether the U.S. NTD Program adheres to this multi-faceted approach. Documents by the Administration maintain the NTD Program is part of a complete package of services the United States provides to improve the health of women and children across sectors.[27] The Administration intends, for example, to expand the provision of drugs that treat STH in children within USAID-supported education programs.[28] Similarly, the Obama Administration underscores the intersection between water and sanitation and categorizes it as a "cross-cutting area" under global health. Nonetheless, in reports to Congress on progress towards advancing global health (through congressional budget justifications, for example) the Administration provides little information about how water and sanitation programs advance global health efforts or how they are integrated within global health projects.

The structure of the FY2013 Foreign Operations budgetary request suggests some separation between these activities. Requests for water programs are made across a variety of accounts, primarily Development Assistance (DA) and Economic Support Fund (ESF). In FY2013, for example, the Administration requested only 12% of water and sanitation funds through the Global Health Programs account and 76% through the DA and ESF accounts. These two accounts support a wide range of governance and economic development activities, which do not typically focus on health objectives.

Despite the limitations of mass drug administration, the U.S. NTD Program focuses almost exclusively on MDA. Administration officials recognize the importance of a comprehensive NTD Program, but maintain that "the directive from Congress was to focus on mass drug administration. [G]iven the limited resources, [MDA] is the most efficient and cost-effective way to control [and] eliminate these diseases."[29] The 113th Congress might debate the merits of applying an intersectoral approach to the NTD Program. Broadening the U.S. approach may not necessarily entail raising spending, but could involve improving the integration of U.S. health and development programs. The 113th Congress could, for example, request information on how key leaders at USAID (e.g., the Deputy of the Global Health Initiative and the Water Coordinator) coordinate their programs.

Strengthening Health Systems

Despite the consistent decline in NTD cases since the turn of the century, weak health systems and conflict in some developing countries continue to hamper efforts to eliminate many NTDs. In the case of human African trypanosomiasis (sleeping sickness), for example, the international community had practically interrupted transmission of the disease in the 1960s.[30] Following the marked drop in cases, the recipient countries failed to maintain sufficient funding levels for ensuring adequate treatment measures and disease surveillance. At the same time, conflict in key areas (Angola, Sudan, and

Uganda) hampered efforts to control the disease as infected individuals fleeing conflict entered areas under which health workers initially arrested the spread of sleeping sickness.[31] Additionally, during fighting, health workers were barred from monitoring some areas. By the 1980s, the disease had reemerged, and by the 1990s, cases were growing dramatically (*Figure 4*).

Resurgence occurred for several reasons, one of the greatest being weak capacity to maintain disease surveillance. Weak veterinary and public health systems limit the ability of several affected countries to enhance NTD programs or maintain them after international support wanes. Many critics of "vertical" or "disease-specific" programs see the poor conditions of health systems in several developing countries as an outcome of the burgeoning investments in vertical disease programs. One argument is that disease-specific efforts divert investments from the very public health systems that are needed to support vertical programs. Supporters of disease-specific initiatives argue, on the other hand, that such activities facilitate dramatic, measurable progress. Advocates of this approach point to dramatic reductions in recent years of deaths associated with HIV/AIDS and malaria. The merits of vertical disease programs have been long debated in the global health community and evidence supports both sides of the debate.

President Obama attempted to reconcile both viewpoints when he launched the Global Health Initiative in 2009. While announcing GHI, the President called for the development of a strategy that integrates health programs (where appropriate); supports primary health systems; and coordinates health activities across U.S. agencies. The initiative did not call for an end to so-called vertical programs. Indeed, the Administration has maintained support for key vertical programs like the President's Emergency Plan for AIDS Relief (PEPFAR), the President's Malaria Initiative (PMI), and the NTD Program.

The sustainability of U.S. global health investments was a central focus in the 112th Congress and will likely be an issue of importance for the next Congress. Should the 113th Congress maintain interest in this area, it may consider sustaining existing reporting requirements on implementation of the GHI, particularly those elements that are aimed at strengthening health systems. Key programs (e.g., Global Disease Detection program) supported by the Centers for Disease Control and Prevention (CDC) that bolster surveillance capacity, for example, could be instrumental in advancing the NTD Program.[32]

Sustaining Advancements

NTD treatments are considered relatively inexpensive to administer (*Table 2)*. The treatment costs are low primarily because pharmaceutical companies donate these drugs for little or no cost. Medicines that are not offered for free are typically sold at subsidized prices ranging between $0.02 and $1.02 per course.[33] When signing the London Declaration, several pharmaceutical companies pledged to maintain or increase donations of NTD treatments through 2020 (*Appendix A*). While these steps have enabled the USAID NTD program—and presumably other global NTD programs—to run at low costs, they also mean that these efforts are heavily reliant upon pharmaceutical companies.

According to one USAID official, "without the drug donations, there really wouldn't be a U.S. Government program."[34] As a result of drug donations, for example, USAID was reportedly able to disseminate NTD treatments valued at over $1 billion for $89 million from FY2006 through FY2011. Furthermore, the agency predicts that within two years, USAID will not have to purchase any more drugs due to pharmaceutical donations.

The extent to which global health programs, in general, and NTD programs, in particular, rely on donor support has been both a boon and a burden to health systems in developing countries. Donor emphasis on key health issues, particularly infectious diseases, has enabled recipient countries to concentrate investments in other areas, particularly primary health care. Foreign investments in tackling infectious diseases have contributed not only to reductions in related fatalities but also in improvements in other health indicators, such as child survival and maternal health. At the same time, many developing countries have become reliant upon donors to fund many major health initiatives. In some cases, ministries of finance have reduced national health budgets when foreign health aid has risen.[35] The reasons for cutting ministry of health budgets can include insufficient capacity to spend substantially larger budgets for a variety of reasons including low staff levels; loan requirements (e.g., requirements by international financing institutions to reduce national spending); or redirected spending on other sectors like education, agriculture, or infrastructure.

Global health experts are now grappling with sustaining and advancing improvements seen over the past several years. Given the substantial contributions made by the U.S. government in this area, resources available for addressing global health challenges may undergo scrutiny as the 113th Congress faces public pressure to resolve growing domestic debt. Congress has exercised increased involvement in shaping global health programs through funding distribution guidelines, spending directives and limitations, and priority-area recommendations. Some argue that congressional spending directives have limited the ability of country teams to tailor programs to in-country needs. Others argue that congressional mandates and recommendations serve to protect critical areas in need of support and encourage the Administration to address health issues that it may not otherwise prioritize. The extent of continual congressional involvement will likely face rigorous debate in the 113th Congress.

APPENDIX A. LONDON DECLARATION: TABLE OF DONOR COMMITMENTS

Table A-1. London Declaration: Table of Donor Commitments

NTD Disease	Activity	Financial Commitment	*Contributor*
Multiple NTDs	Outline disease-specific goals and strategies for control and elimination		World Health Organization (WHO)
	Research and develop new programs and country-specific approaches for combating Guinea worm disease, lymphatic filariasis, river blindness, schistosomiasis, blinding trachoma, visceral leishmaniasis	£195 million 2011-2015	U.K. Department for International Development (DFID)
	Maintain support in over 20 countries; expand support to include Mozambique, Senegal, Cambodia	Build on U.S. $301 million investment since 2006	U.S. Agency for International Development (USAID)
	Overcome barriers to success and address critical gaps to achieve the control and elimination of targeted NTDs by 2020	$363 million over five years	Bill and Melinda Gates Foundation
	Expand work in NTD control and program enhancement	$5 million to selected sites in the Americas and Africa	Mundo Sano
	Country level: build stronger community health systems and integrate NTD elimination and control. Regional level: oversee finances for trust fund to fight river blindness in Africa and partner with other entities to expand trust fund to eliminate or control preventable NTDs in Africa.	Extend financial and technical support	World Bank

Table A-1. (Continued)

NTD Disease	Activity	Financial Commitment	*Contributor*
	Apply WHO recommendations for implementing coordinated NTD plan		Brazil
	Implement fully integrated, multi-sectoral NTD plan; reach full geographic coverage of all endemic areas for lymphatic filariasis, STH, and schistosomiasis; map and reach full geographic coverage of trachoma by 2018; build capacity for surveillance and action to sustain gains from mass drug administration program		Mozambique
	Implement integrated plan to control and eliminate NTDs		Tanzania
	Implement integrated plan to control and eliminate NTDs		Bangladesh
	Consider use of Ivermectin for other NTDs		Merck
	Provide third parties, including Drugs for Neglected Diseases initiative (DNDi), access to selected substances out of compound libraries to find new NTD treatments		Bayer
	Provide third parties, including DNDi, access to selected proprietary compound libraries to develop new medicines for certain NTDs		Bristol-Myers Squibb
	Donate Azithromycin to a study on the potential for the drug to reduce mortality in young children		Pfizer
Blinding Trachoma	Elimination of trachoma in China	$6.9 million	Pfizer
	Continued donation of Azithromycin for blinding trachoma until at least 2020		Lions Clubs International Foundation
Chagas Disease	Double existing annual donation of Nifurtimox to 1 million tablets through 2020		Bayer
	Provide DNDi targeted access to proprietary compound libraries to develop new medicines		Abbot, AstraZeneca, Eisai, GlaxoSmithKline, MSD, Novartis, Pfizer, and Sanofi

NTD Disease	Activity	Financial Commitment	*Contributor*
Guinea worm disease	Fill global funding gap	Gates Foundation ($23.3 million); DFID (£20million); United Arab Emirates ($10 million); Children's Investment Fund Foundation ($6.7 million)	DFID, Gates Foundation, United Arab Emirates, Children's Investment Fund Foundation
Leprosy	Extend existing donation of rifampicin, clofazimine, and dapsone through 2020 in quantities requested by WHO		Novartis
	Organize multi-stakeholder initiative to intensify leprosy control efforts		Novartis
Lymphatic Filariasis	Provide 120 million DEC tablets to WHO for its Global Lymphatic Filariasis Elimination program; ensure a sufficient supply of DEC from 2012 through 2020		Gates Foundation, Eisai, and Sanofi
	Donate 2.2 billion tablets of DEC from 2014-2020		Eisai
	Maintain annual donation of 600 million tablets of Albendazole indefinitely		GlaxoSmithKline
Lymphatic Filariasis and River Blindness (Onchocerciasis)	Repurpose Flubendazole to kill adult worms associated with lymphatic filariasis and river blindness; conduct drug reformulation studies; provide expertise for pre-clinical development and provide technical and supply assistance. If pre-clinical development is successful, Johnson & Johnson will co- fund clinical development; obtain regulatory approval; provide technical support		Abbot, DNDi, Johnson & Johnson, Pfizer
	Provide DNDi with access to proprietary compound libraries to develop new medicines that kill adult worms associated with lymphatic filariasis and river blindness		AstraZeneca, Johnson & Johnson, Novartis, Sanofi
	Increase annual donation of Praziquantel from 25 million to 250 million tablets/year indefinitely		Merck KGaA
	Develop child-friendly formulation of Praziquantel		

Table A-1. (Continued)

NTD Disease	Activity	Financial Commitment	*Contributor*
River Blindness	Maintain unlimited donation of Ivermectin indefinitely		MSD
Schistosomiasis	Provide financial support for a WHO school-based schistomiasis program		Merck KGaA
Sleeping Sickness (Human African Trypanosomia-sis)	Extend existing donations of related treatments through 2020		Sanofi
	Extend existing donations of related treatments through 2020		Bayer
	Provide DNDi with access to proprietary compound libraries to develop new medicines		Abbot, AstraZeneca, Eisai, GlaxoSmith Kline, MSD, Novartis, Pfizer and Sanofi
	Partner with DNDi to develop a new oral drug candidate for sleeping sickness		Sanofi
	Logistical support to ensure drugs reach patients at point of care free of charge		
Soil-Transmitted Helminthiases	Extend donation of 400 million Albendazole tablets/year through 2020		GlaxoSmith Kline
	Extend donation of 200 million Mebendazole tablets/year to 2020		Johnson & Johnson
Visceral Leishmaniasis	Provide DNDi with access to proprietary compound libraries to develop new medicines		Abbot, AstraZeneca, Eisai, Novartis, Pfizer, Sanofi, GlaxoSmith Kline, and MSD
	Partner with DNDi to transform drug currently in trials for Chagas Disease as a new treatment for leishmaniasis		Eisai
	Donate AmBisome for 50,000 patients in South Asia and East Africa from 2012-2017; continue program to offer VL at cost; investigate and invest in technologies and process to reduce cost of Ambisone in resource-limited countries		Gilead
	Develop new training tools for leishmaniasis care for health care providers and patients		Sanofi

Source: Adapted by CRS from Uniting to Combat Neglected Tropical Diseases, Table of Commitments, January 30, 2012, http://www.unitingtocombatntds.org/downloads/press/ntd_event_table_of_commitments.pdf.

APPENDIX B. MAP OF USAID NTD PROGRAM

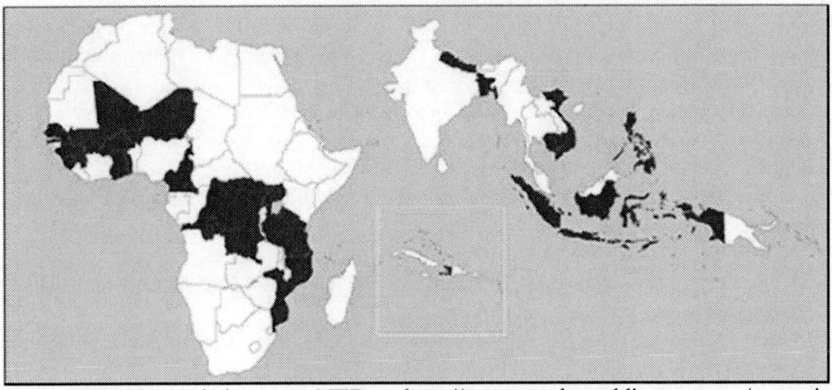

Source: USAID website on NTDs, http://www.neglecteddiseases.gov/countries/index.html, accessed on October 25, 2012.

Notes: The 20 NTD Program countries are Bangladesh, Burkina Faso, Cambodia, Cameroon, Democratic Republic of Congo, Ghana, Guinea, Haiti, Indonesia, Mali, Mozambique, Nepal, Niger, Philippines, Senegal, Sierra Leone, Tanzania, Togo, Uganda, and Vietnam. The countries in which USAID operates can change. In 2011, for example, USAID stopped operations in South Sudan as a result of new investments by another donor focused on NTD control activities in the country.

Figure B-1. NTD Program Countries.

End Notes

[1] For additional background information on NTDs, see CRS Report R41607, Neglected Tropical Diseases: Background, Responses, and Issues for Congress, by Tiaji Salaam-Blyther.

[2] WHO webpage on tropical diseases at http://www.who.int/topics/tropical_diseases/en/.

[3] WHO, Accelerating Work to Overcome the Global Impact of Neglected Tropical Diseases: A Roadmap for Implementation, 2012, p. 16.

[4] WHO, Global Plan to Combat Neglected Tropical Diseases 2008-2015, 2007.

[5] Mass drug administration refers to preemptively treating all people in an affected area without testing to establish individual diagnoses.

[6] Ibid, Accelerating Work to Overcome the Global Impact of Neglected Tropical Diseases: A Roadmap for Implementation, 2012.

[7] Eradicate means to end all transmission of a disease worldwide by exterminating the agent. Eliminate means to reduce transmission of a disease to a predetermined low level (not necessarily zero) with the aim of interrupting the transmission cycle. When elimination is achieved, MDA is no longer necessary and case detection is used to identify individual

cases. Control refers to operations or programs aimed at reducing incidence or prevalence of a disease.

[8] http://www.unitingtocombatntds.org/downloads/press/ntd_event_table_of_commitments.pdf.

[9] Hotez, Peter "Mass Drug Administration and Integrated Control for the World's High-Prevalence Neglected Tropical Diseases," Clinical Pharmacology & Therapeutics, vol. 85, no. 6 (June 2009), pp. 659-664.

[10] For more information on related efforts by these agencies, see CRS Report R41607, Neglected Tropical Diseases: Background, Responses, and Issues for Congress, by Tiaji Salaam-Blyther.

[11] See respective websites of each organization for additional information on their NTD Programs.

[12] Section 593, P.L. 109-102, FY2006 Foreign Operations Appropriations.

[13] See White House, "President Bush Announces New Global Initiative To Combat Neglected Tropical Diseases," press release, February 20, 2008.

[14] For more information on GHI, see CRS Report R41851, U.S. Global Health Assistance: Background and Issues for the 112th Congress, by Tiaji Salaam-Blyther.

[15] USAID et al., Lantos-Hyde United States Government Malaria Strategy, 2009-2014, April 2010.

[16] For more information on U.S. and international efforts to improve access to clean water and sanitation, see CRS Report R42717, Global Access to Clean Drinking Water and Sanitation: U.S. and International Programs, by Tiaji Salaam-Blyther.

[17] See CDC, WASH Away Neglected Tropical Diseases, Activity Summary, June 2010, http://www.cdc.gov/ healthywater/pdf/global/programs/wash-away-ntd-summary.pdf and CDC, WASH Away Neglected Tropical Diseases, Program in Brief, June 2010.

[18] Philip Musgrove and Peter Hotez, "Turning Neglected Tropical Diseases Into Forgotten Maladies," Health Affairs, vol. 28, no. 6 (November/December 2009), p. 1698.

[19] Burton Singer, "Viewpoint by Burton Singer: Bring Back Primary Prevention for Relieving the Burden of NTDs," PLoS Medicine, vol. 7, no. 5 (May 2010), p. e1000255; and TR Burkot et al., "The Argument for Integrating Vector Control with Multiple Drug Administration Campaigns to Ensure Elimination of Lymphatic Filariasis," Filaria Journal, vol. 5, no. 10 (August 2006).

[20] The United Nations (U.N.) General Assembly adopted a declaration in 2000, which among other things, committed member states to advance health development around the world. See, United Nations Millennium Declaration, September 18, 2000, http://www.un.org/ millennium/declaration/ares552e.pdf. Shortly thereafter, delegates developed the Millennium Development Goals (MDGs) to guide attainment of the priorities outlined in the Millennium Declaration. The eight MDGs are: (MDG1) eradicate poverty and hunger, (MDG2) achieve universal primary education, (MDG3) promote gender equality and empower women, (MDG4) reduce child mortality by two-thirds, (MDG5) reduce maternal mortality by two-thirds, (MDG6) combat HIV/AIDS, malaria, and other diseases, (MDG7) ensure environmental sustainability, and (MDG8) develop a global partnership for development. MDG7 includes the water and sanitation targets.

[21] Guy Hutton and Jamie Bartram, Regional and Global Costs of Attaining the Water Supply and Sanitation Target of the Millennium Development Goals, WHO, 2008, p. iv, http://www.who.int/water_sanitation_health/ economic_mdg_global_costing.pdf.

[22] OECD, Aid Activity Database, http://stats.oecd.org/Index.aspx, accessed on July 31, 2012. For more information on U.S. spending on improving global access to water and sanitation, see

CRS Report R42717, Global Access to Clean Drinking Water and Sanitation: U.S. and International Programs, by Tiaji Salaam-Blyther.

[23] Sec. 6, P.L. 109-121.

[24] Personal communication with Chris Holmes, Water Coordinator, USAID, October 19, 2012.

[25] In the early 1900s, the Rockefeller Foundation and its implementing partners combined wide-scale sanitation projects with drug administration and public education to eliminate hookworm infections, which plagued much of the southeastern United States at the time. For more on this approach, see E.A. Alderman et al., The Rockefeller Sanitary Commission for the Eradication of Hookworm Disease (Washington, DC: Offices of the Commission, 1915). This book is available on-line at http://www.archive.org/details/cu31924005710839.

[26] Zoonotic diseases are transmissible under natural conditions from vertebrate animals to humans.

[27] Department of State, Implementation of the Global Health Initiative: Consultation Document, February 2010, p. 20.

[28] Ibid, p. 15.

[29] Emily Wainwright, USAID, Senior Operations Advisor, Neglected Tropical Diseases Program, December 27, 2012.

[30] Pere Simarro et al., "The Human African Trypanosomiasis Control and Surveillance Programme of the World Health Organization 2000-2009: The Way Forward," PLOS Neglected Tropical Diseases, vol. 5, no. 2 (February 2011), p. e1007.

[31] WHO, Control and Surveillance of African Trypanosomiasis, WHO Technical Report Series, Number 881, 1998, p. 43, http://whqlibdoc.who.int/trs/WHO_TRS_881.pdf.

[32] For more information on CDC's global health programs, including GDD, see CRS Report R40239, Centers for Disease Control and Prevention Global Health Programs: FY2001-FY2012 Request, by Tiaji Salaam-Blyther.

[33] WHO, Integrated Control of the Neglected Tropical Diseases: A Neglected Opportunity Ripe for Action, May 2008, p. 3.

[34] Information in this paragraph was compiled from correspondence with Emily Wainwright, USAID, Senior Operations Advisor, Neglected Tropical Diseases Program, December 27, 2012.

[35] Chunling Lu et al., "Public Financing of Health in Developing Countries: A Cross-National Systematic Analysis," The Lancet, vol. 375 (April 17, 2010), pp. 1375-1387.

INDEX

C

D

E

F

G

L

M

N

O

S

T

U

V

W

Y

Z